# Life Lessons from Cancer

By Dr. Keen Babbage and Laura Babbage

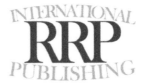

RRP International Publishing LLC
Richmond, Ky.   ·   Greater New Orleans

RRP International LLC, DBA Eugenia Ruth LLC
PO Box 1778,
Richmond, Ky. 40476


www.rrpinternational.org

ISBN-13: 978-0-9898848-1-5

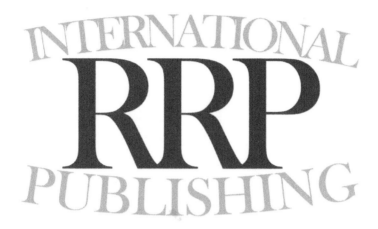

**Previous Books:**

*Son of a Son of a Gambler: Joe McNay 80th Birthday Edition*

*Life Lessons from the Golf Course: The Quest for Spiritual Meaning, Psychological Understanding and Inner Peace through the Game of Golf*

*Life Lessons from the Lottery: Protecting Your Money in a Scary World*

*Wealth Without Wall Street: A Main Street Guide to Making Money*

*Son of a Son of a Gambler: Winners, Losers and What to Do When You Win the Lottery*

**www.rrpinternational.org**

# Dedication

To the remarkable physicians and staff at the University of Kentucky Markey Cancer Center, hospital and clinics. May all the good you do be returned to you many times over.

# Table of Contents

# Foreword

*"We can't afford to be innocent*
*Stand up and face the enemy*
*It's a do or die situation*
*We will be invincible"*
-Pat Benatar

The contemporary that I never got to meet was Steven Jobs. His career with Apple computers kicked into gear about the same time that I started my business and he was someone I followed avidly. I've read every book, watched every interview and felt like I knew him.

I figured that we would get the chance to meet because Jobs did a terrific job of taking care of himself. He was careful about his diet, did not have bad habits and seemed programmed to live a long life.

I will not meet him. Jobs died from cancer at age 56.

Jobs was one of those reminders that cancer does not always discriminate in where it occurs. After decades of study and trillions of dollars, we really don't know that much about cancer. We know that smoking makes you more prone to lung cancer and there are things in our environment that increase the likelihood of cancer, but we don't know why it hits a person who is doing "everything right."

At age 59, Dr. Keen Babbage is the epitome of doing "everything right." He does not smoke or drink. He has had a lifetime of healthy eating, regular exercise and once walked over 400 miles with a baseball to kick off the beginning of the Cincinnati Reds season. He has never been overweight. He has made regular and religious doctor visits for decades.

In short, he is the last guy that should have cancer sneak up on him.

But it did. He found out the same week that his mother died.

Prostate cancer took my strong, athletic father at age 59. He battled like a warrior, but towards the end, Dad wondered out loud about fairness. He had done everything right and still it was not enough. With the double whammy of losing his mother and finding that he had a rare form of nasal cancer, it would have been easy for Keen to give up. Although he knocked on heaven's door several times, he stayed on this side and eventually made it back to the place he dearly loves: standing in a classroom and teaching.

*Life Lessons from Cancer* is not just about Keen. Laura Babbage, Keen's sister-in-law, and I have been friends since we were in a high school play together. She married Bob Babbage, who was best man in my first wedding and remains one of my closest friends. I know the Babbage family well and feel like they are an extension of my own.

Laura is a registered nurse who served as a high-ranking health care executive and, after a midlife trip through divinity school, is now chaplain at the University of Kentucky Medical Center. She knows her way around the health care system and is a strong-willed personality who does not suffer fools gladly.

Laura is the perfect tag team partner in a fight against cancer. She knows the system, is not afraid to say what is on her mind and does not take no for an answer.

In the war against cancer, "going with the flow" will result in death. Keen and Laura prepared to dig in for a long-term fight.

As Keen notes in the book, cancer will either kill you or you will kill it. Cancer is not interested in peace negotiations or shuttle diplomacy.

Keen's story is a terrific perspective from the view of someone with cancer, but another great story comes from Laura. She is a world-class caregiver and used the website, CaringBridge, to give frequent, if not daily, updates on Keen's treatment and blunt assessments of the situation.

The stark and honest reports, without the slightest bit of sugar coating, let those of us who care about Keen know what was going on. I read them within seconds of their being posted every day. CaringBridge also gave a terrific, day-by-day guideline of what a world-class caregiver would do in treating a loved one. Those posts gave Laura a roadmap when preparing her part of the book.

*Life Lessons from Cancer* is not just the story of a cancer patient and his sister-in-law. It's the story of two extraordinary people who teach lessons that all of us will learn from.

Not just lessons about cancer, but about life. It's a terrific story and I am glad to help them tell it to the world.

Don McNay, CLU, ChFC, MSFS, CSSC
Best-selling author, publisher and syndicated columnist

# Introduction

Perhaps you have always dreamed of writing your own book because you have a compelling story to tell or an idea to share. Maybe there is something you have dreamed about, talked about and even attempted to put into words on paper.

For me, this is not *that* book.

Cancer was never the topic or content of a book I hoped to write or co-author. I am the sister-in-law of Keen, the subject of this book. My husband, Bob, is Keen's older brother. Bob and Keen are the children of the late Judy and Bob, Sr., who divorced when Keen was 12 and Bob 15 years old. Judy, or Nana as we called her after our three children were born, was a single mother who steadfastly and lovingly created as normal a home for her two teenage boys as possible. Bob and Keen, devoted sons and brothers, decided at a young age that in the midst of sorrows and setbacks, they had each other and that was what mattered most.

In October of 2010, at the age of 56, Keen was diagnosed with small cell peri-nasal cancer—a fast-growing cancer that had spread from his nose into his cheek and was beginning to invade his brain. Keen lived alone his entire adult life and took meticulous care of himself, got regular check-ups, ate well, exercised regularly and prayed often. He was, we thought, the last person susceptible to cancer. But cancer has no boundaries.

Our book tells the story of Keen's cancer diagnosis, treatment and life lessons learned along the way. Keen's "Lessons" are interspersed with my chronological "updates" which were posted regularly throughout treatment to a website called CaringBridge. It provided family and friends with regular updates on Keen's condition, sometimes graphic, but always real. Keen said, "I want to be as open as possible about my cancer, maybe it will help someone else who is going through it or will face a similar diagnosis in the future." That's Keen, always the teacher.

One of the things that struck me as I reread the CaringBridge entries was how many times I used exclamation points when writing updates. It is only now as I look back over those entries, often written as I sat waiting for a radiation treatment or chemotherapy infusion to finish or for an MRI or CT scan to end, that I realize the enormity of the emotional roller coaster we faced. It is the same for every patient and every family when battling a potentially life-ending illness. When the results of every CT and MRI scan can mean the difference between cancer or no cancer, additional treatments or no other options, life or death, the stakes are so much higher.

Our dear friend Don McNay provided encouragement and support throughout this journey, mentioning Keen's battle with cancer and the CaringBridge website to his many readers in published articles in the *Huffington Post*. Don, author and publisher of several *Life Lessons* books, encouraged Keen to write his story. As editor and publisher, Don arranged Keen's lessons and my posts into this book. Without Don's encouragement, expertise and wisdom, this book would not have been written.

Our hope is that if you or a loved one faces a potentially life-threatening diagnosis, this book will help you navigate through the highs and lows of diagnosis and treatment. It is also a practical resource. There are questions you can modify and ask your health care providers, suggestions for caregivers and loved ones and what to expect if you are the patient. To our friends and family, physicians and caregivers, students and teachers, pastors and prayer warriors who walked this journey with our family, we owe our deepest gratitude.

Laura Babbage, BSN, MA, MDiv.
August 2013

# Life Lesson: Life Hurts

I like to work. As a high school teacher, my work week is usually around 70 hours. I am at school 10 hours each school day. I average one to two hours of school work at home on each school day. I do 10-15 hours of school work each weekend. Family members and friends have advised me for years to work less. I like to work. I thrive on getting results.

In my years as a middle school assistant principal, I averaged 11-12 hours per school day, plus about five hours in the office each weekend and about one to two hours each school night at home. That is also about 70 hours each week. Work can exhaust me, but I return the next day ready for more.

Fighting cancer became my full-time job for four and a half months. My attitude was that fighting cancer was my new job. Each day would have its to-do list which had to be completed. When enough to-do lists had been completed on enough days, cancer could be marked off the list.

I miscalculated. Cancer defied the to-do list method. Cancer cannot be to-do listed like a college research paper or a big project at work or preparations for a family vacation. My training had always been based on the process that harder tasks require harder work which will then produce good results.

With enough hard work, the most difficult and the most complex task can be completed, according to my experience, my training and my education.

In the summer of 2010, I noticed what resembled swelling around my left eye. At a regular session with an eye doctor all the usual tests reported normal numbers. The swelling remained, but all of my usual activities continued with no restrictions. There was no change in my vision, no pain, no headaches, no breathing problem, no bleeding.

A few weeks later, after the school year began, I was on the phone with my sister-in-law. She said, "You sound awful." She was right. My mother had been hospitalized that summer. She then had six weeks of recovery in a nursing home. The combination of taking care of my mother and of teaching was exhausting. I did sound awful.

Based on symptoms I described and on a thorough examination, my doctor treated me for sinusitis. I felt very congested and pressured in the sinus area. The medications had no impact. My approach to this task was to persist until a solution was found so I went to an Ear, Nose and Throat doctor I had seen several months earlier for another reason. I was given a shot and much stronger medicine. No relief. No results.

At the same time in September 2010, my mother, who had recovered enough to leave the nursing home and return to her residence, had to return to the hospital. School continued to absorb 70 hours weekly. Caring for my mother would be given all the time necessary. The commandment says to honor your father and your mother. I intended to obey that.

A return to the Ear, Nose and Throat office on Friday, October 1 would, I thought, result in different medication that would finally cure this worsening problem. The physician's assistant realized something was unusual. She alerted a physician who met with me. We immediately did a CT scan in their office. The scan showed something abnormal in the sinus area. A MRI was quickly scheduled for the following Monday.

I asked the doctor, "How concerned should I be?" He properly replied, "We need to see the MRI results before we know the answer."

That made for an unsettling weekend. My mother was hospitalized and her health was declining rapidly. I had an upcoming MRI to think about. School work had to be done. My response to such intersections of tasks and duties and concerns was to work more, to work harder. Certainly, these circumstances can be overcome by applying more work.

The MRI result led to a referral to a physician who is a cancer specialist. By now, what we would soon know was a cancerous tumor could be seen in my left nostril. The physician removed a tissue sample from that nasal mass. A laboratory would receive that for analysis.

My nose, from the place where the tissue sample had been extracted, bled. A lot. I had to go see my mother at the hospital. The bleeding would stop, then start, then get worse. A physician's assistant who helped my mother came to check on her and saw me struggling to stop the bleeding. Finally, the bleeding paused. I stayed with my mother for a few hours and then went home to do school work and to nurse my ailing nose.

Work harder Keen. Compress the nose more. Grade the papers. Fix a quick supper. Return calls. Read the mail. Tough days like this just require more work. You can do that. Problems just need enough work thrown at them and people can live happily ever after. My goal was not to be happy. My goals were to take care of my mother, help her get well so she could return home, keep up with all my duties at school and get this sinus problem corrected. A longer to-do list just needed more hours of work done. I like to work. I am used to work. I could work my way through the increasingly intense days of early October 2010. More work always solved problems.

Not this time. Pardon me for a moment, please—as I have to do occasionally, I must go hack up a glob of mucus which is lodged in my throat. Two and a half years after being diagnosed with cancer, two years after being told I was in remission, one of the side effects I cope with is the gagging, strangling glob of hardened, solidified mucus that sticks in my throat until I coax it out. Yuck.

Mother's health declined. Surgery she had to relieve lung blockage and breathing difficulty was extensive and invasive, yet necessary. She was in the most intensive of intensive care. She would improve a little, but not much and not for long. No matter how many hours I shared with her, no matter how much work I did on her behalf to advocate for her health care, she was declining. She was in intense pain.

Yet each evening when I left my mother she always said, "I will be better tomorrow." Her optimism, courage and faith were inspiring. I would need them in big amounts very soon.

"Keen, as you probably suspected, you have cancer." Life paused on that October 12, 2010 day. What is supposed to be done next? What is supposed to be said next?

My brother and sister-in-law were with me as the doctor presented the diagnosis. My question was "What do we do now?" That is how I have been trained and educated. Work, management and leadership applied correctly will get any task on any to-do list achieved. This is no different, right?

I was told of all the doctors I would see that day. How is it possible that so many people could open their schedule to see the newest cancer patient at the University of Kentucky? That is what they do. That is what their daily to-do list leaves room for.

Before we left the doctor who gave us the diagnosis, we asked the expected questions. Is a second opinion helpful? Should we consider other places for treatment? When would treatments start? What stage of cancer is this?

And one other question. "Will I live through this?" That question seeks a clear answer. Yes or no. No clear answer was available. Sinus cancer is so rare that no statistics were available about recovery rates or length of life post diagnosis and treatment. Different patients react in various ways to the treatments.

The most important question of all—will I live through this—could not be answered for me. I had heard the dreadful diagnosis and I lived through that. There has to be a way to beat this. If the right people do the right work, we can beat this cancer. No guarantee, but there is life and there is meaning in doing the work of fighting cancer.

I would rather have avoided cancer completely and forever. I would rather keep working 70 hour weeks for school. Instead, I would work 168 hour weeks to fight cancer. Pardon me again, please—as I wrote the last sentence my eye had to be mopped up because the radiation treatments destroyed my tear ducts and a subsequent surgery was unable to correct the damage. It looks as if I am always crying. The war against cancer is forever.

Every moment of every day would be devoted to fighting cancer. It sure is good that I like to work. Cancer would seek to exhaust me and to kill me. I will see to weaken it and kill it. This will be more and harder work than my life has known. I thought there were decades of hard work which I could point to as a signature of my life prior to October 2010. All of that work combined is less than it has taken to fight cancer.

*       *       *

Life hurts. I was fortunate to have little or no physical pain at first during the start of the three months of chemotherapy and radiation treatments. Then, after a few weeks, I could not eat or drink. It was too painful to swallow. For 10 days I was hospitalized with pneumonia, a vicious infection, nuclear strength diarrhea, dehydration and related complications. I was too sick for treatments during part of the hospitalization. The pain increased. How could I be getting worse if I was receiving medical treatments?

During the two years after treatments ended, there are pains, plural, daily. New pains still emerge occasionally and join the already established pains. Cancer is unfair, brutal, wicked, evil and sneaky.

These new pains have no cure. They often have no explanation. They seek to do what the cancer did not do. They seek to defeat me. They seek to destroy me. They seek to kill as much of my life as they can.

These pains are kidding themselves. What's an occasional pain when you have been through two and a half years of war with cancer? The answer is not much. Life hurts each day. For the past two years my life has had new hurts added continuously. All I know to do is push through the pain. The pains are not treatable by medical science. They are treated with the human spirit to prevail.

Beyond physical pain, what emotional pains can cancer cause? Sadness. Agony. Despair. Frustration. Disappointment. Anger. Unhappiness. Melancholy. Sorrow. And others.

For me, the response was regret. At age 56, I had much more left to achieve. Knowing that cancer could kill me brought a strong sense of regret. I had anticipated much more living. The thought of life ending before my life's work was completed temporarily filled me with regret. Then regret was replaced with stronger resolve.

Not knowing whether I would live or die, I had to embrace life, fight for life and resolve to prevail.

# The Diagnosis

The phone call came from 4,200 miles away. It was late in the afternoon, a yellow gold sun was setting over the lush green hillside of this small Tuscan town and the cell phone connection was clear. The strain in Bob's voice was evident as soon as he said hello. There was no small talk. Bob was at the hospital with his mother where he had been staying almost continuously for the past 24 hours, and things were not going well. On my last visit with Judy, or Nana as we all called her after the birth of her first grandchild 23 years earlier, less than 10 days earlier she seemed in good spirits and was still holding her own in her assisted living apartment. Now she was in the hospital in critical condition and Bob said, "If the doctors can't stop the bleeding with this last procedure, Mom won't survive the night, it's not good." With deep sadness in his voice and after a long sigh, he continued, "And, Laura, there is one more thing," he paused long enough for me to know that whatever came next was equally as bad as what I had just heard, "Keen has cancer."

You always remember where you were when awful, unspeakable tragedies happen. I was in the break room at work, getting my second cup of tea when I just happened to look over at the television. It was an unusually cold January morning in 1986 at Cape Canaveral, Florida where the Space Shuttle *Challenger* had just launched. Although coverage for space ship launches was not something the general public tuned in to much anymore, this one was big. There was a gifted teacher on board, Christa McAuliffe, a woman of slight build with a huge smile who was selected from among hundreds of applicants to travel with the astronauts into outer space. She had spent many months preparing the lesson plans she would teach from outer space to children all over the world, re-igniting a love for all things space and science.

The astronauts and the teacher boarded the shuttle early that morning. All the final safety checks were made and liftoff was flawless. The camera panned to the family members and close friends who were seated in bleachers at an appropriately safe distance from blast off, but with a bird's eye view of the history-making event. They all cheered as the shuttle cleared the launch pad.

But just 73 seconds after the *Challenger* became airborne, something went terribly wrong. My eyes now glued to the television, I watched with curiosity and then surprise and then horror. There was a plume of white smoke, darting out in an eerily gruesome crook neck formation. The shuttle had broken apart, exploded into two pieces, before the viewing eyes of all the schoolchildren, Christa's students included, and parents and family and the whole world who had tuned in to see this historic launch. In the midst of white smoke, with one part of the shuttle headed in one direction and the other piece moving in another, there was a collective, worldwide gasp.

We learned later that the "O" ring failed—it could not withstand the cold temperature, allowing pressurized hot gas to reach the fuel tank and ultimately cause the breakup of the orbiter. All seven crew members died that day. Christa McAuliffe never had a chance to teach the first lesson from space. Setting down my teacup on the lunch table, I went to find other staff members; surely this was not what it appeared to be. Surely.

Hearing Bob speak the words "cancer" and "Keen" in the same sentence produced the same kind of suspended disbelief; surely you did not just say what I thought I just heard. It was day four of my five day cycling trip through Tuscany, a 50th birthday adventure that had been planned for almost two years. With the phone pressed up close to my ear, there was a warm late afternoon breeze blowing through the small reception area of this quaint boutique hotel in southern Italy, a welcome cooling off from the blistering sun of midday.

I stood motionless in the undersized reception area of the hotel that would be home for just one night as we were scheduled to ride to our final destination, Sienna, in the morning. There was enough room for a reception desk on one side and a few chairs on the other and the already cramped area was filling up with other guests talking in a variety of foreign languages. There were large wooden doors opened wide on either end. I walked toward the rear door, needing more air, a little quiet and a moment to take in the news. "Tell me more," I said. Bob explained in as much detail as possible, none of which satisfied me. "Keen is here at the hospital with Mom, but he can't go in to see her because his nose is bleeding so badly that he has filled up a hospital towel with blood. He had a biopsy done today of the inside of his nose and they have sent it away for analysis. It is bad Laura, really bad, that is all we know."

Bob and Keen were camped out in a waiting room on the fifth floor of the hospital where they had been staying with their mother. She was very sick, bleeding internally and the doctors were having difficulty locating the source of the bleeding and so stopping it wasn't possible. There was one more option, the doctor explained, but if they were not successful, even if I could take the Concorde, I would not get home in time for my final goodbyes. It was ironic that both mother and son would have similar symptoms of a much more ominous problem. Nana bleeding internally and Keen externally, both suffering.

More devoted sons would be difficult to find. Bob called his mother every evening and Keen visited his mother at her assisted living apartment almost daily, attending to her needs as if she were his child. "You don't have to do this for me," Nana would say. And Keen's response was always the same, "How many times did you take of care of me when I was sick? How many meals did you prepare and feed to me? How many diapers of mine did you change?"

The boys' devotion to their mother began at an early age. When Judy became a single parent, her boys were just 12 and 15 years old. In the mid 1960s in the small town of Lexington, Kentucky, where everyone seemed to know each other, divorce was uncommon; it was not something Judy or her boys openly discussed. One day their father was there and the next day he was gone. It would be six years before the boys reconnected with their absent father. Although he lived less than 10 miles away, it might just as well have been the other side of the planet. In time, Judy went to work full-time as the secretary at Central Christian Church, where she would remain an active and engaged member her entire adult life, totaling almost 60 years. At the same time, Bob was entering high school and Keen began middle school seeking answers for what were now very different questions about their futures. It was a "new normal" for this family as they struggled, each in their own way, to find some balance and peace in this adjusted family system. At a critical point in the lives of her boys, Judy became mother and father, homemaker and breadwinner, soother and one needing to be soothed. Her boys became fiercely independent, unwilling to burden their struggling mother with their own seemingly insignificant needs and fears. Judy's parents, who lived in Richmond, Kentucky, who had been such a source of love and devotion to their only child and her boys, took on an even larger role in the life of this now delicate family system.

Keen, who had been the quiet, bookish son, began to find his voice. He had overcome a speech impediment as a pre-teen and was now learning to navigate a new role in his family without the guidance of a father. Bob dove head first into high school. He began writing for the school newspaper and poured himself into academics as never before. Keen began to dabble in sports and later joined the football team where he played tackle. Both boys were determined to find a way through their pain and find success wherever they could. Life lessons learned during those years were never forgotten. Through their struggle and pain, this family bonded together in new, often unspoken ways, taking on roles in the family that would carry them into young adulthood and beyond.

After Judy died, Keen and I were cleaning out her apartment. The discovery of more than three dozen tissue boxes and enough toilet paper for a year prompted the comment, "I think you expected your mother to live to be 100 years old," I said to Keen laughing at the usually frugal son buying with seeming abandon. "I bought more supplies every time they were on sale," he said and then added thoughtfully, "She needed them." I should have known. But I am getting ahead of myself.

The doctors were able to stop Nana's internal bleeding, at least temporarily. I rode my bike to Sienna, Italy and joined the cycling group for a celebratory dinner on the last night of our trip. In the pre-dawn darkness, I took a cab to a neighboring town where I boarded a plane for the long flight home, consumed with questions and emotions that left me unsettled and anxious. Sleep-deprived and travel worn, Bob met me at the airport and took me directly to the hospital. "Thank God all my children are home, don't ever go that far away again," Nana said with relief in her voice as I made my way to her bedside. We learned that she had widespread abdominal cancer that was not treatable given her fragile health. So although the bleeding had been stopped, at least for the time being, the pain was intense. Nana was dying, and she knew it. As our family gathered around her hospital bed, the nurse entered to ask questions about her medical history. When she came to the question about Nana's immunizations, the nurse asked whether or not she would like to receive her annual flu shot. Without missing a beat Nana said, "Why would I want that? I'm dying for heaven's sake." It was a painfully sobering response that prompted laughter all around the room. It was confirmation that Nana knew her time on earth was growing shorter by the day.

Nana had made all the preparations for her death many years before. She had planned for her death almost as vigilantly as she had lived her life. We all knew the location of the large manila envelope that contained the arrangements for her funeral and burial, obituary and final wishes. Bob said to his mother, "We don't want you to suffer, so the doctors are working to keep you comfortable, that's our goal." We hoped and prayed to get her a bed on the inpatient Hospice Unit. We uttered a prayer of gratitude when, a few days later, a bed became available.

Keen, Bob and I left the hospital long enough to meet with the cancer specialist, Dr. Susanne Arnold, a family friend and a gifted cancer doctor. It was in the afternoon on Tuesday, October 12th that we rode together to the University of Kentucky Markey Cancer Center. It was our first visit to Markey, a place that would become all too familiar to our family over the next four and half months of doctor appointments and cancer treatments. Dr. Arnold had the results of Keen's biopsy.

Shortly after we arrived we were escorted to a treatment room complete with a large computer screen and keyboard. We waited with a certain sense of dread as Dr. Arnold entered the room. After brief greetings, Dr. Arnold told us that Keen had small cell peri-nasal cancer. It was unusual in that it was not the type of cell the doctors expected to see. Typically the slower growing squamous cell is found with cancers in this area. Keed had the more aggressive, small-cell type. We were told it was malignant, but treatable. Cancers of the head and neck are staged or defined differently than cancers in other parts of the body. Keen had a stage 4B cancer. That meant the cancer had extended beyond a localized area, but had not metastasized to other parts of his body—that was good news, the best of the worst news you could hear. Dr. Arnold scheduled Keen for chemotherapy that very week on Thursday. She also scheduled an appointment with the radiation oncologist, who would talk to us more about the plan for radiation. Dr. Arnold reminded us we were welcome to get a second opinion, but after talking with her colleagues, the team agreed that the best and most effective course of treatment was a combination of chemotherapy and radiation. Because of the aggressive nature of the cancer, the sooner Keen began treatment, the better.

We sat in stunned silence. Questions collided in our minds: How, why, when? Keen took meticulous care of his health and had been seeing a number of doctors over the past three months with a persistent "sinus infection," but there was no indication from any of his doctors that the problem was anything more than a recalcitrant infection. After a few minutes, Keen spoke. He asked all the questions that come to you when you when you first hear the words "cancer," "fast growing," "malignant," "chemotherapy" and "radiation" with your name inserted as the subject. Dr. Arnold patiently and with gentleness and professionalism answered every question with as much detail and honesty as she could. After all the questions had been asked and answered, Keen asked what Bob and I thought. Certainly there were other places in the country to get opinions, but we knew Dr. Arnold and we trusted her opinion. We knew that time was our enemy. We wanted her to lead the effort to cure Keen of this cancer.

After each of us weighed in Keen said, "Let's begin the fight immediately."

# Life Lesson: This is Not a Temporary Battle. This is a Forever War.

"I am sick of being sick and tired of being tired."

I spoke those honest, discouraging, frustrating words to a cancer doctor in April 2011, which was three months after my treatments had ended. This was also three months after all signs of cancer and the tumor were gone.

My brain was thinking, "If the cancer is gone and if the tumor is gone, certainly I should be feeling strong, fit, energetic and vibrant again." Wrong. Very wrong.

I was back at work, but that endeavor fully depleted my energy daily. Bedtime was 7:00 p.m. not by choice, but by the insistence of my weary body. Why was I not feeling better? Why was I unable to exercise? Why did I feel sick, weak, limited each day?

"We put you through a lot. The chemotherapy and radiation treatments put the cancer in remission, but your body was put through a severe ordeal. It is very common to feel as sick and tired as you do."

I had no desire to be common. Cancer acted to kill me. Cancer, so far, had lost. I was still alive, but I was not fully living. Would it ever get better? Would I ever regain full health, full activity, full fitness, full energy levels?

No doctor could answer those questions because each patient is unique and each recovery unfolds with time revealing answers on an unpredictable schedule.

During the summer of 2011, I felt somewhat better. I made myself start exercising. I could do about 10% of what I once did. I longed for the other 90%, but I knew that 10% was a start, a gift, a foundation to build on.

By the fall of 2011 I realized that the progress had stopped. I continued to exercise, but the length of time and the physical challenges I could master were decreasing. I could not break past some very minimal exercise amounts.

I slept poorly because my radiated mouth and throat would scream after about 3-4 hours of sleep with a level of dryness that is found in deserts, summer and planets which have never had any water. Any progress in fitness and energy had reached a plateau.

The plateau was discouraging. Declining from the plateau was worse. During 2012, I noticed further reduction in exercise endurance, overall energy and my hope that someday I would return to the health, fitness and energy levels I knew before cancer.

In April 2013, I again said to a cancer doctor, "I am sick of being sick and tired of being tired." The sympathy and empathy extended to me were genuine; however, the facts could not be changed. My body might improve in the next three, five, eight years. It might not. Cancer could return, but even if cancer never returned, my pre-cancer health, fitness and energy were gone, probably forever.

I never thought that would be the reality I face daily. I always expected complete healing and total recovery.

I am very sick of being sick. I am very tired of being tired. Waking up at 2:00 a.m. with a parched mouth, tongue and throat is cancer's way of taunting me as it seeks to claim a partial victory.

I need a half hour each morning to get my body through an unpleasant routine which addresses throat, mouth, tongue, nostril, eye and ear abnormality. About two hours after I wake up and get to work, I am in a setting where I am still sick and tired, but I have to push through those facts and do my job. I never feel good. I always feel bad or worse. Work makes so many demands on me that my sick and tired body is not allowed any attention.

So far work has been good medicine. It forces me to do activities as if I felt good and had energy. I do wonder how long my mind will be able to overrule my body as the mind says work and the body automatically obeys because it is used to working. The day approaches when this sick and tired body will say to my determined, persistent, usually optimistic mind—no more.

That has not happened yet, but previews of it make occasional appearances. What's more, I am perplexed and frustrated because the sick and tired condition is all day, every day. The sick and tired condition is getting worse. Doctors have no solutions because there are no medical solutions.

What can I do? Begin a new tactic in the perpetual war against cancer. What is the new tactic? Rise above. What does that mean? It means that I will do something each day that rises above my level of sick, tired and encourages someone else who is sick, tired, weary, discouraged, defeated, struggling, searching, without hope, needing encouragement, hungry, alone or otherwise suffering.

Being perpetually sick and tired need not make me miss the perpetual opportunities to do something good for someone else. I can be sick, tired and of no use to anyone or I can be sick, tired and kind to someone. Cancer acts to make me of no use.

My reply to cancer is there is no use in you trying to make me of no use. I'm still alive. I still think. I still care. I still hope. I still matter.

I will arise above. Once again cancer, you lose.

There is no adequate medicine available for the sicknesses I face daily in year three of the forever war against cancer. There are no sufficient treatments available. Surgery has been tried and will be tried again as a possible way to lessen some side effects of the cancer, of the tumor, of chemotherapy and of radiation.

Perhaps sick is not the most accurate word. Being sick is addressed with medical actions that eliminate the sickness. Physically, I feel bad or awful every day. It's as if weights are attached to me and I must carry 50 pounds of burdens. It's as if I just completed a running marathon overnight, every night and wake up exhausted, sore and depleted.

It is also knowing that each day will be no better and probably worse than the prior day. My body is injured and cannot fully heal from the injury. The body has been permanently injured and, as can happen with a physical abnormality, other injuries can follow as one physical weakness causes another part of the body to act, move, function abnormally. There are injuries that do not physically heal.

It forces me to rely on the non-physical parts of life to rise above the limits of the physical part of my life. Physically, I am weak, weary, depleted, low energy and unable to improve. The body has been so damaged that it cannot correct itself.

The body can be encouraged by, led by and at least partially compensated for with the heart, the mind and the soul. Within the cancer patient are inner resources which can rise above the physical difficulties.

I tell myself each morning as the body complains when I awaken, rise from this bed. Get up now because cancer acts to immobilize you. Move. Take the first step. Make yourself do what the body has no interest in doing. The heart, mind and soul say get up. The body will follow that command if the heart, mind and soul insist clearly and compassionately.

My heart, mind and soul are not sick. They sometimes feel frustration as today is more difficult than yesterday or as a day ends with the certainty that tomorrow will be worse than today was.

Such is the war, the forever, perpetual, wicked war which cancer declares daily on the patient. I am not doing as well in some parts of the physical war as I hoped, but the highest priority in the physical war—the cancer and the tumor are gone—has been a victory for over two years.

The mental, the emotional, the faith parts of the war I can win daily, I must win daily. They are the parts I can control.

I am sick of being physically sick. I am tired of being physically tired. The physical reality is that I have been, am now and will continue to be physically sick and physically tired.

Because of that I must have the maximum health, fitness and energy in my heart, mind and soul. My heart, mind and soul can rise above the physical. They have to. There is no other choice.

\*       \*       \*

Today is April 1, 2013. I am 59 years old today. Cancer acted to do all it could to prevent this birthday. Having lost in that attempt, cancer will act to do everything possible to prevent my 60th birthday.

Today I will spend the morning at the University of Kentucky medical center. An expert audiologist will measure my hearing. Chemotherapy damaged my hearing and for a year I have worn hearing aids. My guess is that the hearing has declined further, but the test will tell whether my conclusion is accurate or not.

Later in the morning I will have a CT scan and an MRI. Those tests were done every three months until now. It has been six months since the last CT scan and MRI. The tests are not difficult to endure, but they do challenge your attitude.

The intravenous process is bothersome and always communicates that I am in a hospital. The tunnels you lie in for the tests can be intimidating and awkward. I spend the tunnel time in prayer because being in the tunnel of the CT scan or MRI machine causes any cancer survivor to wonder if they have cancer again. I will be optimistic and hopeful. In four hours these tests will be over. Still, I am concerned and apprehensive. Those occasional headaches of the past few months—could they be signs of cancer, part two?

On a delightful side note, today the professional baseball season celebrates Opening Day in Cincinnati, Ohio. I love that city. I cherish Opening Day. Travel with me to Opening Day in Cincinnati, Ohio in 1980.

When I finished college, I moved to the Northern Kentucky and Cincinnati, Ohio area to work for the Procter & Gamble Company. That outstanding, successful, accomplished company sets the standard for respectable business practices and has been consistently rated as one of the most admired companies in the nation.

My plan had always been to become a teacher, but the unexpected opportunity to work in advertising for the nation's most successful consumer goods manufacturer and marketer was compelling. To do that only 80 miles north of my Lexington, Kentucky hometown was additionally convincing.

I had four fantastic years with the Procter & Gamble Company. My colleagues at that company exemplified work ethic, integrity, honor, competence and creativity. I am twice the educator and twice the person I would have been without the P & G years.

One of my company colleagues was a board member of the Cincinnati area March of Dimes. I was looking for a volunteer opportunity so I could get involved with the community. My colleague put me in touch with the March of Dimes. That led to a once-in-a-lifetime adventure.

The March of Dimes was planning their Spring 1980 Super Walk fundraising event. Many people would get sponsors to financially support them for participating in the Super Walk. I attended a meeting during which the goal was to create ways to promote the Super Walk.

What could the March of Dimes do with the Cincinnati Reds became our question? People in the Cincinnati area love the Reds. As a child one of my favorite events for our family was to travel to Cincinnati and see a Reds game. I collected baseball cards as a child. I listened to Reds games for years. I shared the hope that the Reds and the March of Dimes could team up. The unexpected joy to me was that I would get to be part of the team.

The idea that our brainstorming group created was to suggest to the Reds that someone walk to Cincinnati from a distant city carrying the baseball which would be used to start the season. This would promote Opening Day and the Super Walk.

Events moved rapidly. The Reds approved the idea and suggested St. Louis, Missouri as the starting point of the walk because the sporting goods company that made baseballs for the major league teams was located in St. Louis. Imagine that—someone would walk from St. Louis to Cincinnati carrying a baseball, arrive on Opening Day at the Reds baseball stadium, give the baseball to the March of Dimes poster child who would throw out the ball to a Reds player and begin the season.

I offered to be person who would do that walk. My offer was accepted. Two months of training prepared me for the physical demands of walking 430 miles over two March and April weeks in 1980. Nothing could prepare me for the abundant acts of kindness and encouragement from people in northern Kentucky, from people in Cincinnati, from Procter & Gamble colleagues, from family, from friends, from people in St. Louis, from people in many towns or cities between St. Louis and Cincinnati.

The walk was a joy. The 430 miles were filled with adventures. The schedule brought me to Opening Day exactly on time. The baseball had arrived. The poster child's throw was perfect. The Reds won the game. There was much to be thankful for. The memories of those two weeks are still pure joy.

When I endure days like today, when cancer forces me to go through a hearing test, a CT scan, an MRI test and receive intravenous contrast as part of the CT and MRI, I think of wonderful days from the past. I think again that the way to overpower cancer's actions to end my life is to live a productive, meaningful, good life.

In 1980, I never gave cancer one thought. In 1980, I never gave death one thought. In the years since October 2010, I have thought of cancer, the war against cancer and the impact of cancer on me every day. I have thought of death often knowing that I was at death's door.

In 1980, I was not walking 430 miles from St. Louis to Cincinnati so I could tell cancer 30 years later, "You cannot take away from me what I have already done, cancer. You may impact my future, but you cannot reduce my past."

Now, I do think in such terms. Cancer acted mightily to kill me. Cancer still acts to kill me. Cancer has wounded me and wants to worsen the wounds. Cancer wants to return. Today's tests could show that I am still in remission or could show that cancer has returned.

The challenge is to make the most of each day, to do the most good each day, to help someone each day, to encourage someone each day, to make a difference each day, to achieve the most each day. We have today. We do not know about tomorrow.

The number of days remaining in my life is unknown. That is true for every person. Being alive today is known. What I make of this day, right here, right now is up to me. What I make of this day, right here, right now is not up to cancer.

While with the medical experts this morning, I interacted with them in hopes that the quality of their day would be enhanced. I expressed appreciation for their expertise and help. I asked questions and learned from their knowledge as they applied their insights to inform me. There were some smiles and some laughs.

I would rather not have to get stuck so intravenous material can enter my body. I would rather not lie in the MRI tunnel for 30 minutes amid bizarre noises as various beams penetrate my head and neck. I would rather not have the strange feeling that comes when the contrast flows through the tube into vein. The hours of procedures this morning were bothersome in some ways, but in other ways were marvels of modern medicine. I choose to be thankful for the marvels. That is my choice. Cancer cannot take that away from me unless I let it. I will not let cancer do that.

*       *       *

"Dr. Babbage, I'm calling from your eye doctor's office. We need you to see the neuro-opthamologist you have seen before. They had a cancellation for Monday at 10:15 a.m. in the morning so we scheduled you for that. Otherwise it would be June before you could get an appointment."

Today is Wednesday, April 3, 2012. The school district where I teach is on spring break this week. I spent all of Monday morning having medical tests as part of the on-going follow-up to monitor whether cancer has returned and to measure if the hearing damage has worsened.

The phone message today from the eye doctor's office is bad news for many reasons. The doctor himself left another message. How often does that happen and, when it does occur, how often is it bad news? I would guess that it happens rarely and that when it does occur it is usually to communicate bad news.

On the day I was diagnosed with cancer, the radiation expert emphasized how seriously close the tumor was to my optic nerve. Without saying "Keen, you could be blinded by this ordeal" he made it clear that he was extremely concerned about my vision. No optic nerve damage has been noticed so far. Am I going to be told that vision is now damaged two years after treatments stopped? Am I to be told that cancer is at war with me in a new, diabolical, fiendish, perverse, infernal way?

Tomorrow I meet with that same expert radiation physician. He will explain to me what the CT scan and the MRI from two days ago reveal. Is the cancer still in remission? Is there a new tumor? Is there new cancer?

The fact that I need to see the eye specialist urgently is not good. I saw him several times until I was released as his patient one year ago. The concluding statement was "you would return only as needed." It is needed now.

I have so much planned for the five high school classes I teach to do this coming Monday. I will have to get a substitute teacher, but I will go to school, do my work until the minute I have to leave for the doctor and then return to school immediately after finishing with the doctor.

Bothersome thoughts fill my mind. Will my vision decline? Will I be able to see the rest of my life? Will I be able to see well enough to drive, to work, to read, to function? Do I need to learn Braille soon? I would like to block those thoughts. I would like to prevent those thoughts. I would like to delete those thoughts. Yet those thoughts linger.

As I listened to the messages from the eye doctor and from his colleague, my stomach felt sick instantly. It is almost time for supper. I suddenly have no appetite.

Does this mean that I have to retire at the end of this school year? It is an option, but it is not ideal. Working in public education for one, two or three more years is my intention. There is more work to do. The work exhausts me, but I still get good results. Retiring at age 59 is ahead of the preferred schedule. Will that decision be made for me, be forced upon me?

Soon after hearing the phone messages this afternoon, I quickly prayed. My Christian faith tells me to ask for healing and that is what I did. I will pray, pray more, keep praying for healing, for the doctors to have wisdom, for my students to work hard and behave well whenever I have to be away from school and for other people who face the difficulties which life includes, be it cancer, hunger, blindness, other illnesses and much more.

My life hurts right now in ways it has not hurt for over two years. Cancer never paid any attention to the declaration of remission. Cancer never stopped fighting this war against me. I think I have continued to fight, but I realize that cancer just acted to expand the war with a new offensive. The war never ends. Never.

Cancer, since you must insist on a new offensive I insist on a more potent counter-offensive. Cancer, you lost two and a half years ago. You will lose this time.

The eye doctor just returned my call which was in response to the message he left. There is some swelling in the optic nerve of the left eye. I asked him the exact question I asked an Ear, Nose and Throat doctor in October 2010: "How concerned should I be?" His reply was a quick and confident "not." He further explained that this condition was caught early, can be treated and sometimes corrects itself. That was reassuring. I still have no appetite.

I will fight against this newest offensive. Doctors will join in the fight. Family and friends will enter this part of the fight. Faith is already recruited, trained and at work. I would rather not have this escalation, but it has begun and reality must be confronted.

This is a reminder to the cancer patient that cancer fights a pervasive war against all parts of the patient's life. Fighting cancer is not a temporary battle. It is a forever war. I already knew that cancer is 100% evil, but now I know it is worse than that. I would be ashamed to use the language that describes what cancer is. I will not let cancer cause me to speak outside of my G-rated vocabulary. Let's settle on this—cancer is evil multiplied by wicked multiplied by immoral multiplied by rotten multiplied by villainous multiplied by savage multiplied by inhumane multiplied by barbarous multiplied by torturous. Such is the enemy in this forever war.

April 4, 2013 did bring some mixed news. "No change. They look fine. Except for one area; it might be nothing. We'll check again soon." That was the answer to my question posed to two cancer physicians: "What did the CT and MRI from Monday show?" No change is the best possible result. It means nothing new in the tumor or cancer categories was noticed. It means I have been in remission for a little over two years. The fight is forever.

I will have another CT scan and MRI in late May 2013 to see what the one area is doing. Still, "no change" is further confirmation that there is much to be thankful for. Those doctors also told me that most of the side effects of treatment could get worse, may never get better or, if they improve, it will be a minimal amount over many years, perhaps five to 10 years.

They agreed that the treatments I received were "brutal," yet there was no option. A brutally invasive disease had to be attacked with a brutally potent treatment plan which goes after cancer and which destroys healthy tissue and cells in the path to the cancer. That is reality. These side effects are reality. Coping with them is my constant reality.

The April 8, 2013 very unexpected appointment with the neuro-opthamalogist is confirmation that the war rages. This war is much more intense, complex, lingering and difficult than I originally realized. It will continue. It will get worse.

# Nana's Prayer

Nana arrived at the inpatient Hospice unit and it was all hands on deck. The staff was efficient and helpful, always kind and gentle. She was in pain and our goal was to get Nana relief. I held her in my arms, her head now completely gray was nestled against my chest as I gently rubbed her aching back with my hands. "Does this help?" I asked. "Yes, that feels good," she said, but her strained face and tense body betrayed her words. "Let's get you something to help with the pain," I said. Nana knew the end was near. She wanted to be awake and alert, but she also needed to get her pain under control. The two goals were mutually exclusive. Her nurse injected morphine into her IV and slowly the strain on Nana's face and forehead began to fade after so many days of fighting. She became more still and calm, as the pain that had made a home in her back and neck and stomach over the past week began to leave her body. She rested peacefully for the first time in many days.

We decided not to tell Judy about Keen's cancer diagnosis. As Keen prayed with Nana just before his biopsy he said, "Mom, I am going to pray a very special prayer for myself and all I want you to do when it is over is to say Amen. Can you do that?" She nodded in agreement, knowing this was not like all the other prayers Keen prayed at her bedside. After Keen finished Nana said, "Amen," and then paused, surely feeling the gravity of the prayer, and added with as much devotion as any mother ever has, "PLEASE God, Amen."

After Keen's biopsy Bob kept a constant bedside vigil, talking to his mom about his work and life, praying with her and for her. He held her hand and reminded his mother of all the ways she had cared for him over his life. It was a precious gift of time to sit at her bedside, sometimes silent, sometimes praying. When she appeared to be asleep, he would open his computer screen and answer a few emails. Inevitably when he did, she would open her eyes and ask about his work. Bob would share some of the stories of the day and Nana would close her eyes again, satisfied for the chance to hear about her elder son's life and work. In less than a week, the doctor would order a constant morphine drip to keep Nana's pain under control. After that, she was never fully conscious again.

The day after our meeting with Dr. Arnold, Keen went back to work, to the high school where he teaches 10th, 11th and 12th grade students American History and Political Science. It was anything but normal. Keen calmly shared the news of his diagnosis with the administrators, secretaries, fellow teachers, librarians and all his students, "I have sinus cancer and will need to take some time off to get treatment," Keen said. There were questions and some tears, "Is it curable?" "Will you be back?" "When will you be back?" "How did it happen?" Keen answered all the questions honestly and with as much information as he had. Keen later said, "I wanted to be open and honest, perhaps there is a student who has battled something like this, or will face a similar battle in the future." Keen was always the teacher. In reflecting on that day Keen confessed, "It was the hardest day of my teaching career...it was the hardest thing I have ever done."

We made the decision that one of us would be with Keen for every doctor's appointment and every chemotherapy infusion and radiation treatment; he would never be alone during treatments. If you have never spent a day in a building where chemotherapy is administered, count yourself lucky. Amazing staff, state of the art medicines, great snacks, clean restrooms, comfy chairs, big windows, warm blankets, well-stocked refrigerators, special parking, but even if it had been the Taj Mahal, it is not a place you want to find yourself.

On the first day of his three day regimen of chemotherapy, I parked the car in the lot reserved for those receiving cancer treatments. Before getting out of the car we sat for a moment, steeling ourselves for what lay ahead. We held hands and Keen offered a prayer, the first of many we would pray together before we walked into the Markey Cancer Center for his life saving treatments. The battle had begun. Keen and I walked apprehensively, but with great determination into the building. "I want to be a help to those who are caring for so many sick patients. If anyone can learn anything from me, I want them to," Keen said with the same resolve he practiced everyday in the classroom. Keen, always the teacher.

Big brother Bob bought little brother Keen his first mobile phone, an iPhone, and much to our surprise, Keen took a great interest in learning to use it. He became an expert at texting saying, "I can see why my students like their phones so much," adding, "But the classroom is no place for a cell phone." Keen had made a list of everyone he wanted to contact, key spiritual comrades who he wanted to enlist as soon as possible in his "fight against cancer."

"This is a war that will be won with prayer," Keen said. We spent that first day of chemotherapy, 10 hours in total, texting, calling and making lists of all the people Keen wanted to contact. The next two days of chemotherapy were similar. Keen endured the first of many needle sticks, and every nurse and phlebotomist said the same thing, "My you have great veins." It was a foreboding of sorts, as the weeks of sticks morphed into months the very thought of another needle stick was almost as grueling as the stick itself. But Keen wanted nothing to do with a "PICC" line, a peripherally inserted central catheter, which would have provided a longer lasting access point for the nurses to use to inject his chemotherapy without making another needle stick. "You mean I would have to walk around with a needle sticking out of my arm?" Keen said. "No thank you. We will keep doing it this way."

In an effort to keep family and friends, colleagues and students updated on Keen's treatments and progress we started a "CaringBridge" post. The first entry was made on Thursday, October 14, 2010, Keen's first day of treatment.

# Thursday, October 14, 2010

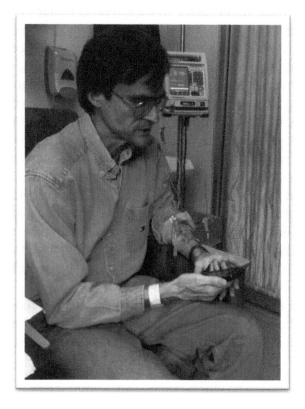

Keen's first day of chemotherapy began today at 8:30am at the Markey Cancer Center. He learned the process of completing the four-by-six inch card where he writes down his name, insurance, date of birth, doctor and a few other particulars, placing the card in the basket and waiting for his name to be called. He was escorted to his "room," which sometimes meant glass doors and three walls and other times was a larger room subdivided by curtains. His room on this day was glass enclosed and included a recliner, IV pole, guest chair and a window large enough where you could recline in the chair and still see outside.

The nurse and pharmacist explained the regime for the day, including the type of chemotherapy, side effects to be aware of and then patiently answered the myriad questions Keen asked. The chemotherapy, by design, is extremely toxic to rapidly producing cancer cells, but because the medicine is not smart enough to recognize only cancer cells, it is also toxic to any fast producing cells in the body. Therefore, the chance of infection increases dramatically 7-10 days after the treatment. Keen will not shake hands or hug friends during treatment, and he will not expose himself to large groups of people. But he will look forward to home-teaching sessions with small groups of students. He will also take special precautions when he visits his mom in the hospital.

After the chemotherapy fluid arrived, the bag containing the liquid was hung on the IV pole and attached to Keen's IV. The fluid would begin its assault on the cancer cells—and on all the rapidly reproducing cells of his body. About an hour into his chemo Keen looked up and said, "My students are making their presentations in class right now...I would love to hear them." We prayed, we made phone calls to the seemingly endless list of friends and ministers whom Keen wanted to keep informed about his cancer treatments. Keen was in a talkative mood, sharing memories about his mom and grandparents saying, "My next book will include a chapter on my cancer." Keen ate and drank when he felt like it, choosing a shortbread cookie and commenting how out of the ordinary it is for him to eat dessert—of course, everything we did today was out of the ordinary.

It was a good day. Tomorrow and the next day we will go back to Markey Cancer Center, complete the four-by-six inch card, wait to be called and begin day two of round one of chemotherapy. We are all adjusting to a new "normal." Thanks for your friendship and prayers—we are so grateful.

# Life Lesson: Alone is Limited, Together is Unlimited

Alone is limited. Part of the fight against cancer must come from the patient. Some aspects of the fight against cancer can come from the patient only. The willingness, the effort, the determination, the drive to battle back against cancer must come continuously from deep within the patient. That patient-driven response to cancer is a necessary weapon in the war versus cancer, but it is not adequate or sufficient.

The cancer patient must team up with family to every extent possible and family must team up with the cancer patient to every extent possible. This is time to abolish, delete, overlook and eliminate any animosities or disagreements. If there are any relatives of a cancer patient, the patient must seek and accept their help. The relatives must offer and provide their unlimited help. Life rarely gets more bluntly serious than when cancer appears.

Recruit friends to be supportive. There are times when the cancer patient is confined to a hospital or to home. The person cannot go out into life for any activities or interaction. Life must come to the cancer patient. For friends, the rule becomes visit, visit more, keep visiting. The patient might be unable to talk, but can listen. Read to them. Talk to them.

The patient may grow weary of listening. Just be there. Share time. Share life. Share togetherness. The patient is suffering. Suffer with the patient.

Some patients may appreciate calls, letters, cards, e-mails or text messages. Communicate in the ways that the patient most appreciates.

Cancer patients can and should initiate communication. Some people may be reluctant to contact a patient for fear of saying something wrong. When the patient makes the first post-cancer diagnosis contact, it can remove the friend's question of "what do I say?"

The medical professionals are well-trained, well-educated, accomplished, helpful people. I experienced no exceptions to that.

Everyone I have met who provides health care for cancer patients sincerely cares about the patient. Reach out to medical experts. Talk to them. Get to know them. Let them get to know you. Become more than health care provider and cancer patient. Bond together as people so you can work together with the extra advantage of sincere mutual concern.

For people of a religious faith, having cancer will put you in a new relationship with your faith. Thoughts can range from "God, why are you doing this to me?" to "God, I thought you loved me. Now this. How can I believe you love me when I have cancer?" to "God, no matter what anyone says, I know this cancer is going to be taken out of me. You won't let this hurt me, will you?" to "God we are in this together, now and always."

What cancer patients believe about God, about faith, about religion will be put to the uncompromising test of hand-to-hand combat during the war with cancer. The presence of cancer should not cause the decline or the removal of your faith. You need your faith now as much or more than at any time in your life.

Do not let cancer separate you from faith, family or friends. Because of cancer, you need more strength than ever from faith, family and friends. Reach out for, receive and accept that strength.

Fighting cancer is not an individual one-on-one encounter. You need an unlimited arsenal of cancer fighting weapons. No one person has the complete arsenal. The combination of faith, family and friends can help complete the arsenal. The outcome is not assured to the fully equipped team of cancer patient, faith, family and friends. The outcome of a solitary soldier alone taking on cancer is more certain and is less favorable.

Alone is limited. Together is unlimited. Fighting cancer is not the time or the place for a solitary, individual, singular resistance.

A cancer patient who is accustomed to being a rugged individual who alone has overcome many obstacles, who alone began a successful business, who alone salvaged a declining local charity, who never asked anyone for help, may think that the same approach will work in confronting cancer.

It will not work. Cancer is a unique obstacle, competitor and foe. There are medical experts whose entire career is devoted to cancer research, cancer treatment, cancer diagnosis, cancer patient health care and they have questions and difficulties despite working closely with their colleagues. If cancer is a challenge to teams of cancer experts, it is more than a challenge to each individual cancer patient.

Your business competitor seeks to take sales from you. Cancer acts to take your life from you.

A charity whose donations are declining needs your advertising, promotion, marketing and financial guidance. The charity seeks to take your wisdom and some of your money. Cancer acts to take your resilience and all of the rest of your life.

At one point I was so sick and so weak I had to be taken by wheel chair from my hospital room to the radiation treatment room. It was decided that I was too sick and too weak to have radiation treatment that day. How does a person begin to recover from being so drastically sick from multiple causes when he cannot be given the treatment one day for his original sickness? A person begins by accepting the help of others.

A nurse wheeled me to the radiation room and back to the hospital room. A family member encouraged me to trust the doctors to know when would be the best time for the next treatment. My faith told me that this was a disappointment, not a defeat.

My best effort was insufficient to counter the cancer, the damage the treatments were doing to my health, the loss of 35 pounds, the inability to swallow and the mental perplexity that comes when you are too sick to take the treatment that is intended to help you get well.

The response had to be a more intense, a higher quantity, and a deeper quality of help from more people. The response had to include more reliance on faith, family and friends plus more effort from me.

Cancer fights with all it has. The cancer patient must fight back with all he or she has within and with all he or she can be given by faith, family, friends and medical experts. Cancer is not fought one-to-one. Cancer is fought one to everything and every person available. Alone is limited. Together is unlimited.

Cancer does not work alone to kill. One cancer cell does not remain as a single, solitary, by-itself enemy of the patient. Cancer cells multiply. Cancer cells are mutant manufacturers of more cancer cells. They grow. They become more numerous. They team up so their cellular chaos can become stronger.

Fighting cancer does not work alone. The cancer patient is the center of the fight. Other people cannot lead the fight for the patient, yet other people must be involved with the patient in the war against cancer.

In the Bible, Jesus says, "By myself I can do nothing." (John 5:30) The motto of the Commonwealth of Kentucky is, "United we stand. Divided we fall." My grandfather, Keen Johnson, told my brother, Bob, and me about 50 years ago, "Boys, we have to pull for each other." The thoughts of Jesus, of Kentucky and of my grandfather—a follower of Jesus and the 1939-1943 governor of Kentucky—match.

Those thoughts advise the cancer patient to build a strong team to fight collectively and harmoniously against cancer. On the day after I was diagnosed with cancer, I went to a pharmacy to get many anti-nausea medications in anticipation of the chemotherapy treatments which would begin the next day. In the pharmacy was a young lady with the pastor's white collar of an Episcopalian church leader. I walked toward her, introduced myself, said something about cancer and asked for her prayers. We prayed together right then in the aisle of the pharmacy. She promised to continue the prayerful support or, as I like to phrase it, "pray, pray more, keep praying."

During the first chemotherapy session on October 14, 2010, which was two days after my diagnosis, my sister-in-law Laura joined me as she usually would during those sessions. How would we spend those six or more hours while the chemotherapy materials flowed into my cancer ravaged body? We made every possible phone call to friends asking for their prayerful support. We called every church where we knew a pastor, staff member or congregation member to ask for prayerful support.

*       *       *

I cannot swallow any food. I have been eating four or five scrambled eggs daily before going to the 7:30 a.m. radiation treatment. Today, I have forced myself to eat a few small bites of the perfectly cooked scrambled eggs.

No more. The food will not go down my throat. The thought of trying another bite is bothersome, frustrating and quickly rejected. I cannot swallow food. I have no interest in food. My body will be fed radiation instead of food. This is a real problem.

I am still fighting cancer. I am enduring radiation and chemotherapy. My body is under multiple attacks. It is refusing to swallow. What message does that send?

I conclude that little food is needed because I am so inactive. Perhaps since I cannot swallow my body is telling me that, for now, eating is not necessary. How can that be possible? Once the body is invaded by cancer and treatments begin, is the body unable to accept food?

Of course the body needs food, but my mouth, throat and brain rejected food. The physical act of swallowing food simply was not possible. The mental thought of eating also had no appeal. The final few bites of food I did eat caused pain. Chewing hurt. Swallowing had gone from difficult to painful to can't be done so do not attempt and do not think about it.

Certainly I could get my mouth and my throat to accept water. How difficult could it be to swallow water? Very difficult. Occasionally, a portion of a sip would go down. I was going to be under-nourished and under-hydrated, but those realities were of no concern to me. I had no appetite. The thoughts of food or water were so bothersome that I avoided both. My weight plummeted. How could this happen just a few weeks into treatments?

About once a week my weight and vital signs were checked. I was encouraged to keep my weight above 160. Impossible. Having begun at 175 pounds, I was soon at 155 pounds and then at 150. Weak. Weary. Sick. Tired.

One regular check at the radiation doctor's office led to a 23-hour hospitalization following immediate intravenous hydration. The 23 hours became 10 days. The IV did my drinking and eating for me. A surgically implanted feeding tube would be my method of eating for several months.

I was more sick six weeks into treatment than I was when treatments began. I weighed 140 which meant 20 percent of my original 175 pounds had been lost. I had pneumonia, an infection,

Dark Ages plague-type diarrhea and cancer. Stage four cancer.

This catastrophic combination condition began because I could not swallow. I could not swallow because radiation treatment had closed my throat. The radiation treatment was shrinking the cancerous tumor. Did I have to die from other causes as the cancer was being killed? If a cancer patient can beat cancer, shouldn't that give them a total victory?

I did not expect cancer to recruit allies to fight against me from multiple directions. I had understood that this war was against a very aggressive cancerous tumor in my sinus area which had grown to threaten my eyes and to begin invading my brain.

What am I supposed to think when my enemies include cancer, dehydration, massive weight loss, inability to swallow, pneumonia, severe infection, diarrhea that ejects from the body like a liquid missile and the accumulated side effects of radiation plus chemotherapy?

I recall one moment of despair. "I am at my limit" was the thought. I had confidently declared war on cancer only to realize that the enemy list had grown. How does a patient fight multiple battles against multiple enemies in an expanding war?

First, decide to fight more. Use every weapon available. The enemy has multiplied. Your retaliation must multiply more. What was a limit must be pushed back.

For me, fighting back more involved other people. To keep death from entering my hospital room, the plan of attack was to fill the hospital room with life.

Friends and family members were with me more often. My body was near death, but my mind worked and could talk. The parts of me that could function, that could show life, needed to be active and interactive.

Some kind health care providers came to my room and explained it is their job to help patients be as pain-free and comfortable as possible. That perplexed me. Pain was not an important issue. Being near death was the issue. If they were suggesting that I was so near death it was time to take actions to minimize the pain as I approached death, I wanted no part of that. I did not think that I was dying. I knew these circumstances could kill me, but I did not expect them to. Why not?

I have always been taught to tackle problems. Cancer was the biggest problem of my life, but an extra measure of the same can-do approach that I always used would be my response. If cancer was going to kill me, and it clearly was acting to, I would keep the attitude and the response of fight back.

I could not swallow. I could not eat or drink. I was bedridden in a hospital. I was on long-term, indefinite sick leave from work. I had cancer. But I could still think. As long as I could think, I would think that I could get well. My actions to get well followed thinking that I would get well.

The tumor had entered my brain. It was not allowed into my thoughts. I was not involved in wishful thinking. I knew the deadly reality of my condition. I also knew that I was still alive. With each breath I took, cancer lost that moment of battle. With each thought of getting well, cancer lost that moment of battle. With each prayer for my recovery, cancer lost that moment of battle.

I could not swallow food or water. Still, so far, I could swallow the hardest shots cancer had repeatedly hit me with. I began to think that if in the midst of these death-defying conditions I am still living, I would live through this.

Cancer was trying to swallow me. As long as I could think clearly, my thought would be to find a way to get well. Whatever else cancer acts to destroy or seeks to destroy, the cancer patient can control his or her thoughts. Cancer cannot swallow that. It makes cancer gag. Do all you can to gag cancer.

When a person is told, "You have cancer" it sounds like the worst possible news. My experience says that more bad news will follow. Be prepared. When I was diagnosed with cancer I never considered asking if I would be able to swallow in a month. The cancer patient cannot anticipate every specific situation that will be encountered, but it is realistic to expect some new difficulties during the war with cancer. Victories can occur, but they will not be without complications, difficulties, losses and despair.

I could not swallow. There was absolutely nothing I could do to fix that. A feeding tube would have to swallow for me. I had to be thankful for the feeding tube, but every glance at it, touch of it, use of it shouted at me, "Keen, you are very sick. This cancer is causing more problems than you ever expected."

When he was about eight years old, my nephew, Robert, was playing in a baseball game. He was at bat with two strikes against him. He barely fouled off the next pitch. He got an even smaller slice of the pitch after that. The next pitch was smashed into right field as Robert earned a solid base hit.

I asked him after the game, "What were you thinking when you kept getting those little foul tips?" His reply was wise. "I kept thinking that I was going to hit the ball."

Why did he think that? He had practiced a lot. He often hit the ball. Friends and family were encouraging him. With each pitch he concentrated more and was determined more.

I had to keep thinking that someday I would swallow again. Not being able to swallow was a serious problem. It had a solution—the intravenous feeding and the feeding tube. The real enemy was not the inability to swallow. The real enemy was cancer, but perhaps there was an equal or greater enemy—the thought that cancer had more allies than one person could resist.

Solution. Get more allies. Further solution—never let cancer control your thoughts.

Organize a bigger, better and stronger army than cancer has. Think of how to defeat cancer and why to defeat cancer.

When you cannot swallow food or water, swallow the fear and dread that may appear. Deny them. Defeat them.

I could not swallow, but I could fight back. I resolved that the swallowing problem was a setback, not a defeat. I would swallow again, someday. Until then, there was much work to do in the war against cancer.

Even though I never liked it, I had to appreciate and be thankful for the feeding tube. The war against cancer had brought me a new friend—the feeding tube. Now, the feeding tube was on my side. I had a new ally. Take that cancer. I cannot swallow, but my new friend will swallow for me.

I had reached my limit, I thought. Wrong. It was time to remove that line of endurance as the limit. Push the limit back. Go beyond the old limit. Create a new limit. Better yet, remove the limits.

# Friday, October 15, 2010

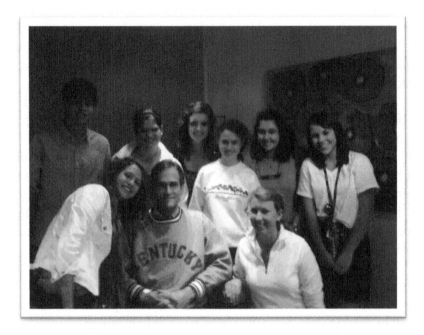

    Keen practically jogged into chemotherapy today. There was a sense of, "Ok, now I know what this is all about and I can do this!" It was his "short" day, just six and a half hours of sitting in a chair, waiting for the IV solution to go into his veins and continue fighting his cancer.

    We talked and laughed and cried some. Keen made some calls on his new iPhone which he is learning very quickly. His first call was to Henry Clay High School. He wanted to be sure the substitute teacher had one last piece of information before starting class today. At one point during treatment, he felt a weird sensation around his heart and thought perhaps the nurses had put something different into his IV. Then he chuckled, reached into his shirt pocket and took out his vibrating cell phone. Every day is new and different.

    At 3 p.m., we went to Great Harvest bakery for a loaf of bread and some cookies. The bread is for Jennifer—his hair stylist and friend. The cookies were for Brian, "my favorite 16-year-old" as he refers to his nephew. "He really likes these, let's get them," Keen said. We took the bread to Jennifer who readily agreed to give Keen a short haircut in preparation for the inevitable hair loss he will experience with treatment.

What Keen didn't know is that we had planned for a small group of his students to support and witness the first "real" haircut (as Bob says) of his life. We gathered around, took pictures and Keen immediately began teaching American History to his students.

He didn't miss a beat. The students gave Keen a card that read, "Fight, Fight more, Keep Fighting."

It is a variation on Keen's constant reminder to his students, "Read, read more, keep reading."

He was touched to the core—everyone was. We are fighting. We plan to win.

# Saturday, October 16, 2010

Keen completed the first round of chemotherapy today. He has 18 days off before he begins round two. Today he read about how cancer fighting drugs came to be as a result of chemical warfare used during WWII. Keen said, "I can incorporate this as I teach about WWII—the students will love it." Keen is always thinking about his students.

As difficult as it is to be confined to a chair receiving treatment for something Keen never expected, it was not the most difficult part of the day. At 5:55 p.m. Nana died. She said her only goal in life was to be a good mother—she said it over and over and over again—and Keen and Bob repeatedly told her, "Well done." The blessing is that Nana did not have to live through Keen's diagnosis and treatment. Now she can walk with him on this journey in a way that she could have never done on earth. For that we are grateful!

Tonight Keen is busy grading papers and preparing for a home study session with some of his students tomorrow afternoon. In the midst of the funeral planning, Keen wants to give his students a chance to review chapters 11-12 before the test. He will teach a little American History and then have a brief lesson on the art of making scrumptious granola bars, the one and only recipe Keen has attempted and perfected over the past 30 years.

Our house is abuzz with life and learning.

# Nana's Goodbye

After day three of round one of Chemo, Keen and I left the hospital. He was weary, but he would have an 18 day reprieve to regain his strength before round two began. It is the first 21 day cycle of chemotherapy. "The effects of chemo are cumulative," Dr Arnold warned. "You will get more tired and experience more symptoms as the treatments progress." On the final day of round one, he sat in his recliner chair for six hours. "They are getting more efficient," Keen said, as we drove directly to the hospital to see Nana. She was nearing the end. Her breathing had slowed. I held Nana's frail body in my arms and whispered in her ear, "I promise to take care of Keen with as much love and gentleness as you would if you could." Keen spoke to Nana from the side of bed, with a mask covering his nose and mouth. With tears in his eyes he said his final goodbyes.

"Do you want to stay a little longer?" I asked, knowing that her days had dwindled to hours. "No we had a schedule, let's stick with the schedule," Keen said. So we left. I had no idea yet how much Keen relied on a schedule; it is how he managed every day of his life and how he would fight the battle against cancer as well. Bob arrived at the hospital at 5 p.m., just as we were leaving and sat by his mother's bedside, speaking softly to her through gentle tears, holding her hand and praying her into the arms of God.

Just before 6 p.m. she quietly slipped away. Bob called us weeping and said, "She's gone." No matter how much you expect death, it's always a surprise. "She waited until I got through my first round of chemo," Keen said from the chair in our family room where he was sitting as tears of gratitude fell from his eyes.

"Yes, she did," I said with as much gentleness as I could. "Yes she did."

Nana's lifelong prayer was that she would never have to bear the sorrow of burying one of her children. That prayer extended to her grandchildren as they came along. In her final days I remembered that prayer and thanked God for that faithfulness to a woman of such deep faith and constant prayer. Nana's death spared her the unbearable burden of watching her son suffer through cancer treatments.

Keen and I returned to the hospital after Nana died. We cried and prayed as we gathered around her hospital bed. Judy's minister of many years arrived to offer prayers and comfort and later our Catholic priest came to offer a prayer with our family. Keen, extremely aware of the warning from his doctors not to risk infection, stood at a safe distance from his mother. He had held her hand and prayed with her so often over the years that he was content to pray from his place in the room. We said our final goodbyes to Nana, thanked the nursing staff who had cared for Nana and our entire family with such concern and gentleness and left the hospital. We had arrived at another "new normal" in our lives that would change us forever—life without Nana.

The prayer that found itself on my lips and making a home in my heart was from Psalm 31, "Into your hands I commend my Spirit." We reluctantly, so reluctantly, returned this woman of great faith and hope and love back into the arms of God from whom she came. There was a celebration in the midst of the sorrow.

# Life Lesson: If You Give Up, You Lose. If You Persist, You are Winning

"I am at my limit." That was not supposed to happen. That was not part of the plan of attack against cancer. If I am at my limit, but the war with cancer has not been won yet, how do I avoid defeat?

It was very perplexing and confusing to me when I heard myself say the words, "I am at my limit." It is not an option to be at my limit because there is more work to do. The treatments have not been completed. The tumor is shrinking, but it has not disappeared. A smaller cancerous tumor is still a cancerous tumor. The tumor is not at its limit. It is still fighting and, while it has been losing, it has not yet fully lost.

If "I am at my limit," does that mean I have nothing left in my heart, mind, body or soul to call upon as we continue this war? On the day in December 2010 when I spoke those words to a beloved pastor, what did I mean?

I did not mean surrender. Being at my limit did not mean that I could not continue the war. I did not mean that cancer had won the war and that continued offensive actions against cancer would be wasted efforts.

I did not mean that I was depressed. When some people suggested that I consider taking anti-depression medications, my response was an emphatic, adamant refusal. Nothing in me was depressed. Nothing in me suggested depression. That was how I saw it. There was no reason to further confuse my body with additional medications as the body was coping with anti-nausea pills, chemotherapy, radiation and intravenous fluids.

"I am at my limit" should have been phrased, "I am at my old limit." I was sicker than I had ever been in my life. I was closer to death than I had ever been in my life. Any boundary or limit I had known in the realm of physical illness had been surpassed and had entered territory that was new to me.

I spoke the words "I am at my limit" to one person only and one time only. After hearing myself speak those words, my mind was filled with questions and analysis.

On a weekend when I had 15 hours of papers to grade, what had I always done if after 15 hours of grading I was not finished? The only answer had been throughout my teaching career—keep grading. I would manage the weekend hours so the work was completed before optional uses of time were considered. Except for church and family, nothing would be done on a weekend until the last paper was graded. Sometimes that meant nothing was done except church, family and grading.

What I anticipated as a 15-hour limit of my grading endurance had to be extended to 16, 17 to 18 hours or whatever the final number had to be.

One of the most memorable lessons in management I was taught occurred when I was 22 years old and a new employee of the Procter & Gamble Company. I answered a question from my boss about the $3 million marketing budget I was managing. Her reply to me was, "That's unacceptable." The message was clear—do not accept what is; rather, make it what it needs to be.

Any limits of endurance, persistence, energy, determination and willingness to fight obstacles that I had prior to cancer were now unacceptable. Cancer was a stronger enemy than I had ever faced. All limits had to be removed. Cancer's wickedness and fury knew no limits. The difficult side effects of cancer treatments knew no limits.

I now realized that as a person who was fighting cancer I had to remove all limits I had ever imposed on myself or that my body was inclined to set.

I cannot run a mile in four minutes. I have never been able to run a mile with any real speed. But I can think of it so vividly that I see myself crossing the finish line in three minutes 59 seconds. I can think beyond the current limits.

My thoughts expanded beyond my prior limits. I was not at my limit. That statement was completely wrong. My thinking had to change. Keen, you are not at your limit. You have reached and extended beyond old limits. Is cancer placing any limit on what it does to you? No. So remove all limits in what you do and how you do it to fight back.

If I stayed within my old limits I would lose. The edge of those limits had insufficient ammunition to slay cancer. I had to surpass those old limits and fight back against cancer with no limits.

In my war with cancer, I never again said or thought "I am at my limit." I prefer to fight cancer with no limits to my counter-offensive.

Cancer forces a cancer patient to do more than find out what you are made of. Cancer forces a cancer patient to find out what he or she needs to be made of and to reconstruct himself or herself accordingly.

Limits? What limits? I do tell my students that everything in class must be G-rated, legal and ethical. My war with cancer was consistent with those principles, but would be far beyond the maximum effort I had ever made for, on or against anything. Fight cancer with no limits. That is how cancer fights you.

*     *     *

One year after I was told that the cancer was in remission I asked one of the cancer physicians who has been with me from the start of this war, "How sick was I?" The answer was, "Without the most aggressive treatments possible, you probably would not be here."

That means I was at death's door and the door was open. The answer came as no surprise. From the day of diagnosis, I knew that the cancer intended to kill me. I knew it was very rare cancer, very aggressive cancer, very determined to cause death cancer. I knew that the treatments were strong enough to kill a very large cancerous tumor. They were strong enough to damage my sick, weak, declining body further.

What prompted my question at the one year after treatment ended mark which was also the end of one year that the cancer was in remission? I was feeling worse. For about three months after treatments ended, I felt stronger day to day and I gained some of the 35 pounds I had lost. Then, the progress stopped. No more weight gain. Minimal appetite. New side effects. Worse conditions of old side effects. What does all this mean?

If the treatments work and there are no signs of cancer, why do I feel so awful and why is everything worse?

Because some wounds in warfare never heal, some other wounds get worse and new wounds that were latent appear. That seems so unfair. It is unfair. It also is reality. Some parts of life will never be what they were before you had cancer. That means some parts of life will never be as good as they were before cancer attacked.

Is it possible for other parts of life to become better? That is completely up to you. Enduring cancer does not automatically make you a better person; however, someone who has endured, survived, defeated cancer has new reasons to maximize the good parts of life which are fully available for new effort, new dedication, new commitment and new results.

# Monday, November 1, 2010

Today was a GREAT day! Keen practically jogged into the radiation department, determined to be one of the patients who brightens the day of all the employees who work at UK. Every Monday after his treatment we meet with the nurses and doctors about his progress and concerns. Last Monday it was good news—the tumor is shrinking, Keen looks and feels better, *but*....His doctor said, *but* we are concerned about the optic nerve as the radiation must be in very close proximity to the nerve that controls vision in order to kill the cancer.

It was a huge but—as we left Keen said, "It is one more thing we have to pray about." I was less controlled saying, "I just want one day when all we get is GOOD news!"

Well, today that prayer was answered! I practically came out of my seat when the doctor said, "The tumor is shrinking—if this keeps up we can look at backing off the radiation and recalibrating the machines to keep away from the optic nerve." It was beyond good news.

And that's not all. In the past week Keen has gained two pounds! He is still three pounds down from where he started, but the scales are moving in the right direction. We meet with the nutritionist later this week to learn more ways to pack in calories and keep him healthy and well fed. It will be a full-time job for Keen to eat—he is up for the task.

Finally, there is one more piece of good news. Every visit Keen asks, "If there is anyone who can learn from my experience, please use me." This week Dr. Marcus Randall, the Director of the Radiation Oncology Department, has taken Keen up on his offer. He is structuring a teaching/learning opportunity for Keen with medical students—this is a real gift and allows Keen, the master teacher, to be both teacher and student.

It was a very good day indeed. We remain grateful for your visits, cards, words of encouragement and prayers. We will continue to fight, fight more and keep fighting until every cancer cell is gone.

# Friday, November 5, 2010

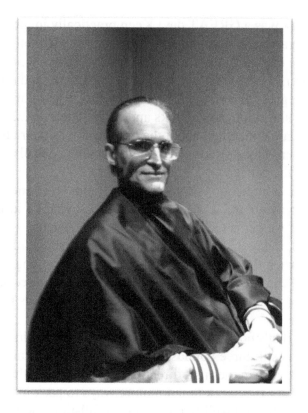

Keen will complete his second round of chemotherapy tomorrow and his second week of radiation ended today. "Everything happens on the schedule they gave us," Keen said as we witnessed his hair loss which began in earnest today. "We better get that haircut. Let's call Jennifer," Keen said with that emphatic tone which causes his eyes to focus intensely accompanied by a slight smile that says, "It's ok."

So we called Jennifer, Keen's hairstylist for over 20 years, who moved heaven and earth to cut his hair today. With shears in her hand and some hesitancy Jennifer said, "It is so hard to cut his beautiful hair, but it will grow back." She also offered, "You just don't know what the new hair will look like, it could be curly!" We laughed heartily and immediately began plotting new hair styles for

Keen as he makes his daily adjustment to a "new normal." The crew cut, slicked back look gives Keen a bit of that movie star appeal, a la Michael Douglas? Regardless, it is one more outward affirmation that the chemo and radiation are doing what they are designed to do—kill cells that divide quickly without the ability to be selective.

And so Keen has begun to experience tasteless food, "but I eat it anyway," he says with a smile. Keen delights in telling the nurses, technicians and doctors that he is eating in ways that he has a hard time imagining. "I had a piece of transparent pie for breakfast yesterday," he said with a chuckle. "Goodness!" he added to convince any doubters that he is working hard to beat this tumor, keeping weight on any way he can.

The results continue to show. Clearly the tumor continues to shrink as evidenced by daily radiation scans and physical changes including better breathing and vision. At his Wednesday appointment with Dr. Arnold, Keen's oncologist, she told Keen with great delight that her original thought of six rounds of chemo could be more like four to six rounds which could potentially get him back in the classroom sooner. Keen smiles, I cry.

Keen's response to his cancer reassures everyone. He asks about each nurse, doctor and technician who treats him. He remembers their stories and the names of their family members. During chemo we call friends to update them on Keen's progress and Keen will say, "Oh, ask about her mother," or "see if ____ passed the exam," or "ask how their trip to _____ went." We joke because "chemo brain" can be a side effect of treatment (temporary forgetfulness), but so far the only person impacted is me! Keen's response is, "Well if we both get it how will we know?" And we laugh.

Keen feels your good thoughts and constant prayers, we all do. Keen's response is pray, pray more, keep praying. And Keen's response is to fight, fight more and keep fighting to beat this cancer.

# Sunday, November 7, 2010

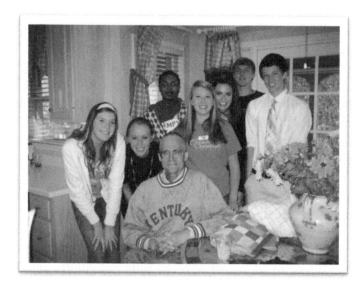

     Keen has a new haircut! He was feeling well enough after his second round of chemo and second week of radiation to have a study session with students today. Keen's spirits are always lifted when students visit. We had snacks, great discussion about the recent elections, questions about US History and updates on fighting cancer. It was a good day.

# Thursday, November 11, 2010

HARD week. This is the third week of radiation and as promised, it is grueling work. Keen is now having difficulty swallowing; his mouth is so sore it hurts to talk. "If it is going to be this way until December, maybe they can put me in a coma and wake me up when it's all over," Keen said, only half in jest.

Today he got pain medicine that helps some. With medication Keen gets some mouth relief which allows him to eat, of all things, mashed potatoes with loads of butter. Mashed potatoes is about all he has been able to get down today—the consistency is right and it does not require chewing, a chore that his mouth cannot take. So we eat mashed potatoes and talk, so long as the pain medicine is working. I have heard some great family stories and Keen's wit and humor have not diminished, even in the midst of these hard days.

Radiation is cumulative, and Keen is halfway through the treatment. Of course, the effects of radiation will last beyond his last treatment—which is good news and bad news. Keen has a second MRI on Monday to see how much the tumor has shrunk and to hopefully limit the radiation field. He had an appointment with the neuro-ophthalmologist who says all vision parameters are normal and unaffected by the cancer—GREAT news!

And so we continue to pray and pray more. Our hope is that Keen will be able to stay well-nourished so he can avoid a temporary feeding tube. We also hope that his pain can be controlled with medication. Today, with some pain meds, Keen helped shop for a birthday present for his nephew, Robert. He even posed for a few pictures of the potential gift—we had a great time at the store.

Keen is still planning on a study session with students this Sunday but plans to take a break from the sessions after this one. Chemo and radiation is like trench warfare—you have to conserve your energy for the big fight. He loves hearing from his students and remains inspired by their work while he is away.

# Friday, November 12, 2010

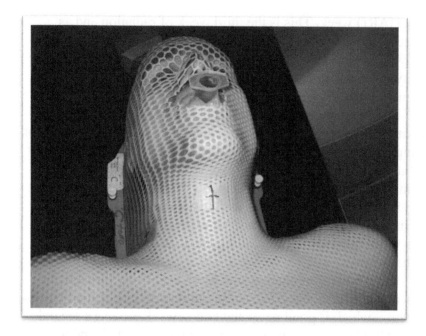

Today is a difficult day at the end of a difficult week—totally normal and completely miserable! However, Keen will begin a pain patch today to keep his pain under control. We also met with the dietician and have some new menu ideas to compliment mashed potatoes! Keen thinks up most of the ideas, always doing the work required to get better. Keen asks great questions and sometimes stumps the caregivers—in that case, everyone learns, one more victory.

Keen said, "I sleep during radiation now," which is amazing given that he has a mask that covers his face and chest and is bolted to the table that slides into the Tomography machine. It is a new schedule for everyone, and we continue to find many things to laugh about along the way.

# Life Lesson: Be Realistic

"You have cancer." When those words are heard, a new reality exists which will impact every part of a cancer patient's life.

Hearing those words, "You have cancer' means that whatever life had been for the cancer patient will never be exactly that way again.

When a physician tells a patient "you have cancer," the doctor is being honest, direct and realistic. The patient now must also be realistic. "I have cancer" is the start of a sentence. "I have cancer and I am declaring total war on cancer" completes the sentence.

Be realistic. That does not mean be pessimistic or fatalistic. That does mean to know the facts of your cancer condition. Know the treatment options. Know why the doctors are recommending one particular treatment plan. Know what to expect during the weeks, months, years of treatment. Of course, different people react to treatments in different ways, but know what data and experience suggest a person with the cancer you have and with the treatment plan you have can expect.

Know what the percentage possibility of survival is. Each day you live is a 100 percent survival rate, but there may be days when all you can do is barely survive. Know if you should expect days like that.

Know what percentage of people with the cancer you have and the treatment plan you have live for one year, three years, five years, 10 years and beyond 10 years.

Know what your insurance will pay for. Know what the doctors and the hospital expect in payments from insurance, from government health care programs which cover you and from you personally.

As soon as I was diagnosed, there was a steady stream of paperwork. The "this is not a bill" statement would arrive almost daily. I kept precise records of those because questions would arise. Several times a duplicate bill arrived for an expense I had already paid because the processing of my payment was slower than the processing of the duplicate bill. Be very realistic about the mountains of paperwork and of accounting work you must keep current. Deal with these as they arrive even though it is a chore and you do not feel like doing it.

Be realistic about what you can do while receiving treatments. Some cancer patients keep working or going to school or fulfilling other duties during their treatment process. Other cancer patients find that the treatments prevent them from doing anything else. I missed four and a half months of work which is more work time than I have missed in three and a half decades of employment. There was no option. I had to be realistic, yet the intention of returning to work was a major incentive to me.

Cancer of any type is serious. Cancer of some types and some degrees of or stages of development are more serious than others. Take cancer very, very seriously. "Oh, they caught it early and not much has to be done" is not the approach to take. "They caught it early which helps, but it needs thorough treatment and very careful monitoring after that" is more realistic.

Think of cancer as the world's most wicked, evil, relentless, invading army which has one goal—to kill you. Cancer does not negotiate or compromise. Cancer fights an all out war. When cancer is in your body, recognize it as an internal terrorist which uses modified guerilla warfare tactics. Cancer does not hit and run. Cancer hits again and keeps hitting. Your treatments must hit cancer harder that cancer is hitting you. That warfare occurs within your body. You will feel every shot fired, explosion ignited, battle waged and counter-attack launched. Be realistic—you are in a war.

There are many cancer survivors. They endured the war and prevailed. Life after cancer is different for them than life was before cancer. The words "life after cancer" are perhaps misleading because I increasingly suspect that even if cancer never returns to my body, my body and my health will never return to what they were prior to cancer. That is reality.

There is honor in your fight against cancer. Fight valiantly, fight vigorously, fight persistently, fight confidently, fight realistically. Other people can be inspired by your fight. Other people can find hope in your hope. Other people can find faith in your faith. Throughout the fight, be realistic. Know the enemy.

When you have a cold or the flu, you do not think of those conditions as an enemy. They are illnesses which, given some time and medication, should be gone on a reasonable schedule. Reasonable means a short time. Gone means fully eliminated. If another cold or another case of the flu hits you later, those could also be resolved.

Cancer is the enemy. Be realistic. Cancer has declared war on you. You are now a soldier in the trench warfare against cancer, yet you must also be an officer, a commander, a general, a leader. There are many troops, officers and other leaders in your army. Keep everyone's total attention and effort on the total war which must be waged against cancer. Keep yourself, your family, your friends, your health care providers optimistic, hopeful, determined, fully concentrated and 100 percent realistic.

The reality of having cancer must be addressed with full acknowledgment of that reality and with full commitment to a total war against cancer. That is reality. In fighting cancer, there is no alternative but to be fully realistic while remaining fully committed to the mission and fully confident in the possibility of victories, including small victories that can occur moment to moment.

Cancer means war. That is reality. Know the reality. Know the enemy. Fight the war. The struggles will be brutal. Injuries, wounds, setbacks will occur. Some days will be awful and other days will be worse. Fight the war.

Cancer is fighting you. That is reality. Fighting back is the new reality of your life. Be realistic. You have no other serious option. The fact is you have cancer. That is reality. Now, from that reality create unprecedented strength, will, hope, confidence and endurance to fight back. Become the realistic cancer warrior that the reality you face requires to you to be.

\*     \*     \*

There were bad days. There were awful days. There were terrible days. There were absolutely disastrous days.

There were zero good days. There were some good moments. There were some good hours. There were no good days.

Why not? Why could there not be any good days? Because at

some point on every day you wonder what is going to go wrong next. Because at some point every day you wonder what part of your body is going to be damaged or change or not function or need help. Because at some point every day you wonder if all of this will ever be over. Because at some point every day you wonder if your reserves of resiliency are depleted.

Because at some point every day you wonder if life will ever be normal again. Because at some point every day you wonder, you question, you think about, you silently or aloud ask—am I going to live through this or am I going to die?

I was able to leave the hospital in early December 2010. I had to have 24 hour per day help for two weeks. I had to be fed through the feeding tube several times daily. I needed help with everything except sitting in a chair and reading. I had more radiation treatments to endure. There would be more chemotherapy when the body was strong enough.

Sitting at home, unable to go to work, unable to drive because of a pain killing/preventing medication patch I wore, needing help with everything, unable to eat, unable to and not interested in trying to swallow anything, needing constant care. Were these good days?

No, but they were better than being in the hospital. They were better than awful or terrible. For a cancer patient, a day that is not awful can be, on a comparative basis, good.

The way you keep score changes when you have cancer. A bad day used to be one with too much work, too many e-mails, too little sleep, too many chores, too many demands on your time, an irritating muscle ache, a hurried lunch and an unfinished to-do list.

Now, a bad day is when you are told you have cancer or when the cancer treatments nearly destroy you, when you keep wondering if you will ever get back to work, when you stare at death.

A day when the treatment has no difficulty, when friends visit, when family members go to chemotherapy with you, when the family dog sits extra close to you all day because he just knows you need some extra care, becomes a day for which a cancer patient is thankful. There becomes a new definition of what a good day is.

Good now means not horrible or awful. Cancer changes your definition of words and your appreciation of the details in life.

# Monday Nov 15, 2010

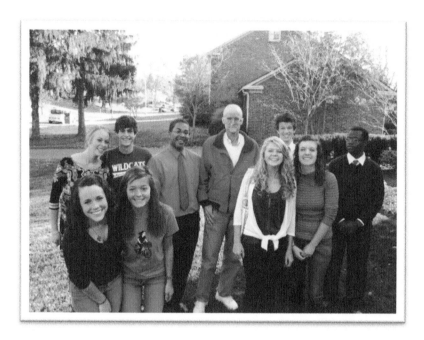

After a difficult week last week (there are more descriptive words I could have chosen), Keen gained 2 pounds this week. It is amazing that we gauge progress by food eaten, weight gained (or lost) and pain managed. Radiation is cumulative and week three was predicted by the experts, but came out of nowhere to the inexperienced cancer patient. What started out as a jog into radiation has morphed into a slow walk, albeit with Keen's unfailing sense of humor.

Keen stays cold most of the time these days and so when I found him in the living room with a blanket over him I asked, "Are you cold?" "No." Unconvinced I touched his hand and said, "You're actually hot, Keen," to which he replied, "Why thank you, Laura!" We laugh a lot.

Keen's students visited yesterday. I will post pictures and a note about that uplifting experience. Keen is having an MRI now and a CT scan tomorrow. We meet with his oncologist and radiation doctors on Thursday when we hope to hear good news.

# Tuesday, Nov 16, 2010

GREAT NEWS!! Keen's oncologist called to say, "I didn't want you to wait until Thursday to hear some good news...the tumor has shrunk significantly...it appears as though the radiation fields can be more limited and we can back off the optic nerve." It was an answer to prayer. Keen's response, "Thanks be to God!" We meet on Thursday with Keen's oncologist and radiation doctors to learn more about the upcoming plans for his treatment based on the results of his MRI and CT scan. Right now we are elated!

There is also good news as Keen continues to talk with various people about how he can be helpful to the learning process at UK. Some of the folks in the Behavioral Sciences area are working on ways Keen can interact with individual and small groups of medical students. Keen says, "I want to help them see how a person with cancer looks and feels in the _____ week of treatment—it will be better than reading about it in the textbook."

It's true. They will see the sunburned look to Keen's face and neck where the radiation is targeted and they can examine his mouth to see the internal effects of the treatments that are life-saving yet painfully difficult to tolerate. He can share how his food intake has been reduced to mashed potatoes and scrambled eggs, and how he experiments with other foods to see what he will be able to eat this week of treatment. There is much to be learned and no one teaches quite as effectively as Keen, using whatever means he has and adapting the "classroom" so learning can occur.

# Thursday, November 18, 2010

Keen is in the top five percent of his class. Dr. Arnold shared this news today as she reviewed the results of the MRI from Monday. "Your progress so far with Chemo and radiation meet or exceed our expectations." Music to our ears. We have a long way to go, but we are thankful for improvements so far. We learned that the cancer is no longer in the frontal lobe of the brain. The tumor has also backed away significantly enough from the optic nerve that the radiation fields will be narrowed to help spare the nerve and, we hope, preserve Keen's vision post radiation.

On the nutrition front, Keen has been told he needs to gain back weight lost. The problem is that the only thing he tastes is the nasty antibiotic crushed up in apple sauce—all food tastes awful. However, today Keen said, "I have an idea...let's stop by Graeters." We shopped for the highest calorie ice cream they make and made a Blizzard out of it. "I don't taste a thing good, but I can get it down...it is even a little soothing to my throat," Keen said. Tomorrow morning breakfast will include five scrambled eggs chased by two scoops of ice cream. Anyone want to join us? Pray, pray more, keep praying.

# Saturday, November 27, 2010

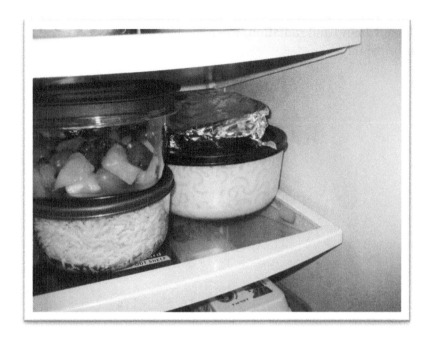

Chemo: Round three, day two. It is a difficult day. Keen is tired and edgy. The thought of two more weeks of radiation and all the side effects is close to overwhelming. Yet the doctors remind us, "It will get better, I promise." Keen has lost more weight. The idea of a temporary feeding tube is the last thing he wants to think about, but it may be the thing he needs right now.

"Call the doctor today, please, so I can ask what to expect these next two weeks of radiation and then afterwards," Keen asked this morning. Knowing what to expect makes dealing with it all somehow manageable. Keen would like to get off his pain patch as soon as possible so he can drive again—you have to give up so much control when you are in cancer treatment that driving again will be a mini victory.

On a lighter note: I opened the refrigerator on Thanksgiving Day and found a small piece of a carrot sitting on the shelf. Confused I asked Keen, "Did you put this carrot here?" Without hesitation he said, "It's Rudy's treat for after supper." Rudy is our dog, who loves Keen. I laugh every time I open the fridge. The picture I will post later today says it all! And, Keen visited with his first medical student yesterday. Morgan asked penetrating questions and saw firsthand what a person looks and feels like who is in the midst of Chemo and radiation. Keen the teacher—it was the best hour of the day.

# Sunday, November 28, 2010

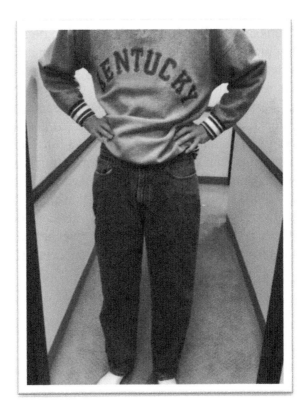

Chemo: Round 3, day 3.

Keen's face, where the radiation beams have been specifically targeted, has gone from a sunburned hue, to tanned, freckled and peeling. Radiation is harsh. Food intake is nearly impossible now—expected but dreaded. His radiation doctor will have a "strategy" for nutrition just as he has had for every problem encountered during this course of treatment. "You would think they would have developed 'strategies' to avoid some of this," Keen the educator says with a look that says, "I would do that for my students." Keen laments to his doctor, "I have gone from tired to practically lethargic." Expected. Check. He has traveled through these stages of treatment with the side effects anticipated.

When asked by his nurses and doctors, "Is there anything

else you need, anything else we can do?" Keen says later, "Can you wake me up in January when this is over?" But he walks through it with impeccable manners and gratitude for everything being done for him.

On Thanksgiving Eve Keen said, "I used to do all my Christmas shopping on this night." With his mask on and dressed for cold we went to the mall. Instead of shopping for everyone else, we bought clothes for Keen. "When was the last time you bought a new pair of jeans," I asked. "I don't know, maybe 20 years ago," Keen answered matter-of-factly adding, "These have worked fine."

Almost two hours later we left the mall a bit weary with a new pair of Levi blue jeans, tan corduroy pants, a thick warm fleece jacket and sweat pants. "Will you wear your new cords to school next semester?" I asked. All I got was a look that said, "You've got to be kidding." Keen wears a tailored suit and tie to school every day of the year. There is seriousness to a suit that matches Keen's intensity in the classroom, one complements and reinforces the other.

# Last bite

Just as we had done each night for the past week, we prepared scrambled eggs, drenched in butter and filled with shredded Colby cheese, thinking of every possible way to get as much protein and fat into this man who was withering away before our very eyes. As he weighed in each week at the doctor's office, before the needle sticks and meeting with the doctor, he wore more clothes, heavier clothes. This particular morning he attempted to weigh in with his coat on, determined that he would not lose one more pound. He looked at me sheepishly when I called it to his attention and that of his nurse. I almost regretted saying it, except for the fact that I knew he had not eaten one bite of anything for the past 24 hours. In fact, he had hardly taken a sip of water. I was worried.

The night before he sat before his plate of eggs, determined to eat, willing himself to eat, but finally, with tears streaming down his face, he said, "You wouldn't think it would be so difficult...I can't do it." Not wanting him to see my eyes fill with tears, I turned away and said, "I have an idea."

We put our coats on and walked to the car. It was our nightly routine to drive to Keen's house to "check on things" as he put it. But there was such a heavy sense of dread hanging over our family on that particular evening that we couldn't even speak. So I plugged in my iPod and turned it to the song "Corner of the Sky," from the Broadway musical, *Pippen*. In the solemn silence we listened as the lead character sang, "Everything has its season, everything has its time, show me a reason and I'll soon show you a rhyme... Rivers belong where they can ramble Eagles belong where they can fly, I've got to be where my spirit can run free, Got to find my corner of the sky."

By the time the refrain played, we were both singing. It was a song that took us back more than 30 years earlier to a hot summer evening in Dayton, Ohio. Keen wanted to spend some time with the woman who had become a serious love interest in his brother's life and so he bought tickets for us to see the musical *Pippen*, which was being performed on the campus of the University of Dayton. Keen was working as an assistant Brand Manager for Procter & Gamble in

Cincinnati, Ohio, his first full-time job after college and I was living in Northern Kentucky. The ride up to Dayton is a blur, but the ride home was filled with excited conversation about the musical; the acting, the music, the choreography, how much we loved every minute of the performance. Years later, as Keen recalled the story of our meeting he would insist, with his dry sense of humor, "I was Laura's first choice, but I was too old for her so she married my older brother."

For those few minutes in the car ride from our home to his, we were transported back to a happier time, a time before needle sticks and chemotherapy, before radiation masks and the slow burn of good tissue and bad in the nose and throat and face. At least for that moment, there was joy.

Each evening we drove to Keen's house to pick up the mail and the newspapers, even though his neighbors had volunteered to take care of those chores. And just as he did every evening, Keen checked every door and every lock in the house. He checked the door to the refrigerator and touched all four burners on the stovetop and opened the door to the oven, even though, in the 22 years he lived in that house, he had never once turned on the stovetop or cooked anything in the oven. Then he walked to the basement that he and his dad had finished many years earlier. After checking the locks on the sliding glass doors that led to the backyard, Keen walked through the laundry room, unlocked the door that leads into the garage and made sure his white Toyota Camry was exactly as he had left it. Satisfied, he locked the door and made his way slowly back up the steps. It was the same routine each evening. I waited silently. After he was assured that the house was secure, he was ready to leave, locking the front door and checking it again before returning to the car. A wet white snow had just begun to fall and the night seemed somehow darker than usual. We drove home in silence.

# Life Lesson: Hope is Real. Magic is Not Real

I was diagnosed with cancer two and a half years ago. The treatments stopped and I was told that the cancer is in remission just over two years ago. After a few months of gaining some strength and a feeling of health, most of the past two years have been times of decline in energy, fitness and overall health. I never feel good, yet I push, prevail and persist.

Today I woke up at 2:53 a.m. I was very thankful. In recent weeks I have been waking up at 12:30 a.m. or 1:14 a.m. so to sleep until 2:53 a.m. was a wonderful gift. Cancer makes you think differently. Before cancer, a 2:53 a.m. wake-up would have been annoying. Now it is something to rejoice about.

As I woke up this morning, there was one very clear thought: I do not feel awful. I felt bad and the morning routine was necessary to help my eyes, mouth, throat and other declining conditions or other cancer treatment side effect collateral damage realities function sufficiently to begin the day.

Still I did not feel awful. I felt bad, but it was bad that could be managed. To not feel awful, to begin the day merely feeling bad, wow, that was truly encouraging. I rejoiced and gave thanks.

What does giving thanks mean? It means I prayerfully, sincerely and meaningfully thanked God that I did not feel awful. Before cancer, I would never have thanked God that I felt simply bad rather than awful. Since the cancer diagnosis, God and I have discussed my health often. Throughout this entire cancer ordeal, for me, faith in God has been the essential foundation of my willingness to fight back against cancer. Faith is very personal, yet to fully explain my experience with cancer, it is vital to include my adventure of faith.

I am a Christian. My parents, grandparents and great-grandparents were Christians. One of my great-grandfathers was a Methodist circuit-riding pastor. My parents read the Bible to my brother and me, prayed with us and went to church with us. I had my questions during the college years and doubts as a young adult, but those were temporary and unfounded.

I believe in God. I believe that Jesus Christ is the Son of God. I also know that cancer almost killed me. I know that cancer will never quit trying to kill me. I know that my health has declined significantly. I also know that I do not feel awful today.

The chemotherapy and radiation treatments I was given did not work any differently because I have faith in God. I worked differently because of my faith in God.

I believe in prayer. My sister-in-law worked with me, especially during those many hours of the chemotherapy treatments and during my 10 death-defying days in the hospital, to ask many people to pray for me. We were blunt. "Keen is sick, very sick. He has a rare and aggressive cancer. Treatments are strong and often. Please pray."

What does it mean when, as a patient who is fighting a deadly illness, hears often, "I am praying for you. Our family is praying for you. Our church is praying for you."

It means that you are not alone. It means that while your body is seriously struggling, your soul is more seriously mounting a counter offensive. Will you survive? That is not known. What is known is that you are fighting back with every possible resource.

Part of the war against cancer for me was impacted by my mother's death a few days after I was diagnosed. Her bold, honorable, faithful, inspiring words guided me. Days before her death she eloquently told her family, "If I die, do not grieve. Rejoice that I lived a good life."

It was possible that cancer would kill me in 2010 or 2011. It did not. Cancer has seriously harmed me and continues to inflict difficulties. One way to defeat cancer is to live a good life in one day allotments. Cancer will forever try to kill me. Today I do not feel awful, so cancer loses today.

When you face cancer, you face the reality of death. One way to outsmart death, no matter the cause of death, is to live a good life. My mother knew that. My mother, a devoted Christian, knew that death was not defeating her because living a good life for 83 years was her victory. Her home now is heaven. She lived a very good life on earth. She lives a glorious eternal life in heaven.

My faith tells me that when I die I will live forever in heaven. Until then, my faith requires me to live a good life of belief, of action, of hope, of caring. Faith sustains me in the war against cancer. When nothing else goes right. When the body is completely overwhelmed, when the mind is perplexed, when the heart is discouraged, the soul can prevail.

The Bible tells me in 2 Timothy 4:7 to fight the good fight, keep the faith and finish the race. Part of the race of my life is to run against cancer. Part of the fight of my life is against cancer. Faith, for me, is the foundation for the fight. Victory is not measured only in how long the fight can be extended, but in how well the fight is fought day to day.

On a day when I do not feel awful I can rejoice, give thanks and tell cancer that it lost that day. On the days I do feel awful I must fight the good fight harder than ever. There is honor in such increased effort. For me, that increased effort is built upon, sustained by and reliant upon faith in God whose Bible says, in Matthew 19:26, "Jesus looked at them and said, 'with man this is impossible, but with God all things are possible.'"

I never would have thought that for God to give me a day of not feeling awful would be a reason to be thankful. It is such a reason. I did not feel awful today. Rejoice. I have been given this day. Rejoice again.

Cancer victims survive the diagnosis. How long a cancer patient survives after that is initially unknown. There is no guarantee about the length of the war against cancer, but that war lasts the rest of the life of the cancer patient.

What is guaranteed is that how the cancer patient fights back against cancer can be determined by the patient. We would rather not have cancer for ourselves or for anyone. Still, cancer exists and for patients, their families and their friends, how we fight back is a new measure of living a good life. For me, the fight began with faith and continues with faith.

*       *       *

I had e-mail recently from a former student. The e-mail arrived on a day that began with me feeling awful. By the time I got to school, I merely felt bad. "Dr. Babbage, you were my teacher five years ago. I never cared much about school until your class. You got me interested in learning. I will graduate from college soon. I am going to be a nurse. Thanks for helping me realize what I could be. You are a great teacher."

The student's timing for that e-mail was perfect. Despite feeling bad, perhaps I could do something on that day which would make a difference for a student, a colleague, a friend, a relative. Part of fighting cancer is a belief that as long as our life continues we can still do good for and with other people. My faith expects that of me and I am thankful for that expectation.

Cancer, I know you are going to act to make me feel awful tomorrow. I will cope with that then. For today, I simply feel bad which, for me, is just wonderful. My faith tells me that the essential variable is not how I feel, but that "This is the day the Lord has made, let us rejoice and be glad in it." (Psalm 118:24)

I cannot change the fact that I am a cancer patient. I cannot change the fact that cancer has injured me. I cannot change the fact that I feel bad today. But I can fight the good fight. Keep the faith and continue running the race. OK, I will walk the race very slowly, but each step will be with faith knowing that I never walk alone. That makes it possible to walk through anything.

*     *     *

Chemotherapy will cause the cancer patient's hair to fall out. I was told to consider two options: one, go ahead and cut the hair off completely, or two, have it cut much shorter than usual now and then when the falling out gets worse, have it cut off completely.

I chose the second option. The haircut became quite an event with family members, some of my students and a lot of pictures. There were smiles and laughs. Not much was said about cancer. The haircut was necessary because of cancer so that was obvious.

When the hair falls out you no longer look like yourself. The mirror becomes an ally of cancer, if you let it. There is a difference between, "Look at me. My hair is gone. I never looked this bad in my life" and "Look at me. I can still stand up and see myself in the mirror."

The war against cancer is not about hair, but because hair coming out is such a visible indication of cancer and cancer treatment, it is part of the war. On a day when you do not feel awful, but you look the opposite of how you used to look, it is hard to avoid feeling awful about how your looks have changed.

The hair falling out is discouraging and disappointing. Cancer's total package of evil includes unkind, but not detrimental to health, impact such as the loss of hair.

Cancer can kill you. Being without hair cannot kill you. Concentrate on fighting cancer. Losing hair can cause an unnecessary distraction from the real enemy. When the chemotherapy stops, the hair will return. Of vastly greater importance is to improve enough so chemotherapy can stop. Kill the cancer then you and your hair can team up again later.

Recently I saw a picture of me when I was in the hospital. Morbidly sick. Emaciated. No hair. I did not recognize the person in the picture as myself until I studied it very closely for about 10-15 seconds. I almost asked, "Who is that?"

If fighting cancer can be so devastating that you do not resemble yourself, then that confirms how gravely serious cancer is. If possible, think beyond the cancer-caused appearance. The war is against cancer. Some of the related skirmishes may matter, but deserve nothing beyond what they really merit which is minimal.

If you gain a sensible view of priorities as you lose your hair, you are outsmarting cancer. Cancer has no brain. The cancer patient does. Continually put that brain to good use.

# Tuesday Nov 30, 2010

Just when you think it can't get worse, it does. "The battle against cancer just became a war," Keen said. He has been admitted to Markey Cancer center for a 23 hour stay for fluids and pain control. Everything he puts in his mouth turns to mucus—eating and drinking, even ice chips, present not only a physical reaction but a psychological barrier that is just as strong. We are hopeful that the surgeons will be able to place the feeding tube while he is here but if not it will be done this week.

There is less laughter now, fewer walks, and more rest. "What can I expect?" Keen asked the radiation doctor. "The last two weeks of radiation are difficult, but the two weeks after that will be the most difficult, then you will slowly begin to feel better." Keen takes it all in, asks more questions attempting to understand what "more difficult" and "most difficult" might look and feel like. How can it get worse? I try not to imagine.

We are already planning to repeat the holidays that Keen misses. Thanksgiving in April, Christmas in May and of course the celebration at Henry Clay High School when Keen returns to the classroom sometime next semester. For right now, however, we take a day at a time.

In the midst of all the pain Keen continues to enjoy the time he spends with students; writing college letters of recommendation, texting and visiting. And in spite of the battle he is in with cancer, he stays busy. Keen's 12th book came out last week—*The Extreme Principle: What Works Best, What Matters Most* (rowmaneducation.com). It is dedicated to his students at Henry Clay High School. He read it cover to cover the day it arrived. And he sent his 13th book to the publisher a month ahead of schedule. It should be out by April. When asked about his next book Keen says, "I think I'll take a break from writing for awhile." Good plan! Thank you for the ways you support us. The war is on—Keen fights and prays and we all cry some.

# Wednesday, Dec 1, 2010

My early morning text from Keen said, "Radiation at 7:30 per Dr. Shah. Is it January yet? I am really eager to get to 2011 ASAP." Keen's assessment of last night at Markey was, "fair." The doctors ask questions and give instructions, the nurses and support staff make suggestions and offer comfort measures. Keen rests and receives IV fluids. The plan is to get a feeding tube today so he can regain his strength. We have laughed this morning and have new resolve to win this war. Thanks for the prayers, food, support and messages.

Keen asks for prayer this morning for complete healing. The prayers need to be doubled because December will be twice as hard as November.

# Thursday, Dec 2, 2010

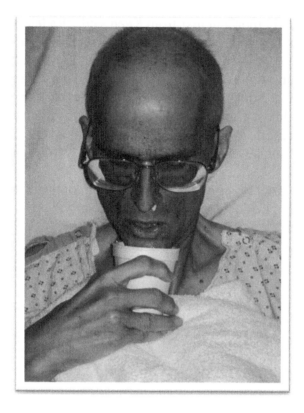

SUCCESS! The procedure to place the feeding tube was successful and uneventful, words we love to hear. Keen waited 24 hours before receiving his first tube feeding; it is going in now. His spirits are already lifted. Yesterday he got hiccups. Not a pleasant thing after having your stomach punctured to accept a feeding tube. So the doctors suggested medicine, but Keen said, "Get me a glass of water please and fill it three fourths full." I started laughing immediately saying, "You aren't going to do that 'drink the water from the opposite side of the cup' are you?" I got that look, half smile, half frown that says, "Watch and learn." Well, it worked, temporarily anyway, but it was the best medicine of the day.

Keen will stay in the hospital until they see how he tolerates the tube feedings. Right now he is weak and his throat hurts so he doesn't talk much. We hope to have him home this weekend. Thanks for all your encouragement and prayers. These are hard days but it will get better—the doctors remind us daily of that fact.

# Saturday, Dec 4, 2010

Rough night. Keen's pain is difficult to control and the tube feedings have caused diarrhea so they needed to be stopped for the time being. The doctors and nurses at Markey work diligently to find the correct mixture of medicines that will alleviate Keen's symptoms and get him back on the road to recovery. In the meantime, we continue Keen's practice of reading five Psalms a day and one Proverb. There is great comfort in the scriptures, especially in the midst of such suffering. Pray that this bump in the road will be overcome quickly so we can get Keen home with us, strong and able to continue treatment.

*     *     *

We now know why Keen has felt so badly—he has pneumonia. The good news is that it is very treatable. The CT scan showed that his feeding tube is fine. The doctor will change the type of formula to help eliminate the diarrhea and re-start the tube feedings this afternoon. He should begin feeling better in a couple of days. This is a set-back but not insurmountable by any means. Keen is resting comfortably right now.

# A Difficult Day

It was an especially difficult day. Keen had been in the hospital almost one week and was showing no signs of getting stronger or better. He was coughing up mucus and becoming more lethargic by the day. The doctors ran more tests and ordered a chest x-ray. Keen was diagnosed with pneumonia. Although it was good to learn that these new symptoms were treatable, there were no shortcuts in the healing process. To make matter worse, Keen had six more treatments before he received the full dose of radiation that his doctors had prescribed in order to kill his cancer. In spite of the pneumonia, Keen was taken by wheelchair to his daily radiation appointment on the ground floor of the Markey Cancer Center. Pristine floors and walls, complete with millions of dollars worth of equipment that rival NASA space shuttles, fill the ground floor of Markey. Keen was immediately wheeled to a treatment room outfitted with a gigantic tomography machine where his previous 29 treatments had been administered.

The efficient, experienced staff who operates the massive machinery took gentle care of Keen as he arrived, sensing the somber mood and anticipated acceleration of his symptoms. Keen, with his hospital gown now engulfing his withered frame, took the tongue protector from the technician with a sense of dread. There were no smiles or kind words, no enthusiasm or teachable moments, he knew the routine and that included opening his raw and achingly sore mouth wide enough to accept the golf ball-sized tongue protector (known as an obturator) or treatment would be cancelled. One more disappointment on top of so many seemed hard to fathom.

He made one attempt after another to open his mouth wide enough to accept the obturator, refusing to give up, wanting so badly to get the next radiation treatment knowing it could make a difference in this now macabre fight against cancer. As he struggled to open his mouth, with determination so strong that his hands shook, tears began to fall softly against his cheek as he finally conceded, "I just can't do it." There were no words left to speak. The gravity of the moment elicited only silence. I turned away, determined to remain strong in spite of this setback, wiping away my tears as the technicians helped Keen back into his wheelchair. I wondered, "How much more can this man take?"

After arriving back in his hospital bed, lying so still with barely enough mass to notice a body among the sheets and blankets, it was difficult to know if Keen was alive or dead, save for the slight up and down movements of the blankets from his breathing . I turned away from his bed and noticed that a soft white snow had begun to fall, adding to the accumulation on the ground and covered walkway joining Markey to the University Hospital. Tears now pooling in my eyes, I sat silently in the vinyl recliner in the corner of the darkened room wondering if this was how it would end. I prayed for relief and comfort for this man who had already endured so much.

At that very moment a good friend of many years walked through the door with a small bag in her hand. She took one look at me and then at Keen and through our tears she whispered, "There were days when my husband was so sick with cancer treatments that he couldn't lift his head off his pillow. I have seen people more sick than Keen—he *can* recover, he *will* recover. Remember that." And with that she hugged me and pressed a bag of chocolates, honey sticks and Lavender- Chamomile tea in my hands. "Drink this and you will feel better," she said. The warm tea with honey was delicious, but her visit was the perfect antidote to caregiver heartache.

I learned that day that caregivers need caregivers too.

# Sunday, Dec 5, 2010

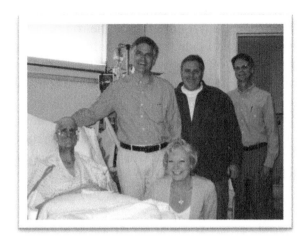

What a difference a day makes!! Keen is beginning the process of recovering from these treatment setbacks. The night nurse was joyful over the changes from her two nights with Keen. And he has a request of all CaringBridge compatriots. Today at 2:30 p.m. we will gather to pray with Keen. He has written out the prayer below that he wants everyone to pray with us at that time (God will hear regardless of when you pray, of course).

\*     \*     \*

*Dear God,*
*You are in control. We do not fully understand all you are doing, but we believe in all you are doing. In recent weeks, it seems to us that everything that can go wrong has gone wrong. Now, we ask in the name of Jesus that from this moment on in the war against cancer, the tumor and all the side effects, pneumonia and everything else that our healing results are not merely good but are perfect as our Heavenly Father is perfect.*

\*     \*     \*

Keen had a good day. His pain is more controlled and he is able to do more for himself. We had a prayer service in Keen's room today, at his request, and we read the scriptures he chose and the prayer he wrote. Each of us shared our own prayer—it was good medicine. This evening, after completing the routine of care he gets, he flexed his muscle and made that face, half smile half grin and said, "It's gone!" I told him that when he walks all the way to the nurses' station and back I'll play the *Rocky* theme song. We both laughed.

We are hoping tomorrow will be a day of steady improvement. Keen will likely be at the hospital for another week. It is not a bad thing as he has no idea what the last week of radiation will hold—which he hopes to resume tomorrow.

# Monday, Dec 6, 2010

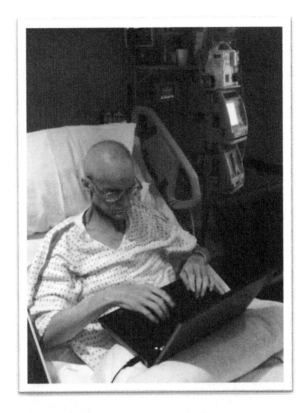

Oh my, it has been a very good day! I will attach a picture of Keen at his computer—a sight to behold given the last week. And not only that, but Keen is renaming all the hospital equipment. Of his "incentive spirometer" he quips, "there is no incentive!" We all laugh. A breathing machine is a more appropriate description to which the doctors readily agree.

Radiation has been postponed until the pneumonia has a chance to resolve—a disappointment, but not a deal breaker we are quickly reminded. This break allows some of the normal tissue a chance to heal and that may make swallowing a possibility again in the near future.

It was a good day and we are hopeful that tomorrow will be even better. Thanks for all you are doing to help make this diagnosis and treatment manageable. We remind all the doctors that as grateful as we are for all they are doing, we would rather not be here. They nod in agreement.

*     *     *

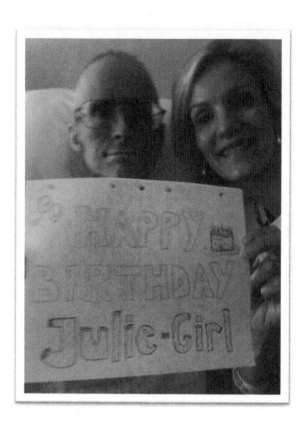

Oh, I almost forgot to say that Keen called his favorite niece Julie to wish her a happy 19th birthday today. He agreed to celebrate it with her when she finishes her exams and comes home for winter break. So much to look forward to.

# Tuesday, Dec 7, 2010

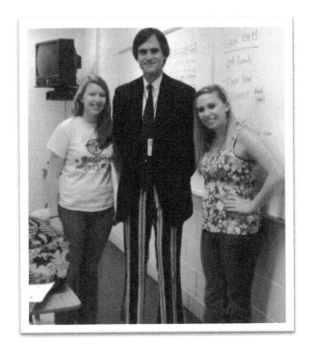

It is always the little things that mean so much when you are a patient in the hospital. Keen walked from his room down the hall and back to his room. It was an occasion for cheering given the past week. The really great news is that he completed another day of radiation today. One down and six to go. It prompted a few high fives and a tear or two. "Now, if you can just drink six to eight ounces of water every hour," I said. "It sounds so simple doesn't it?" was Keen's response. When everything tastes like run-off from a mine the next six ounces of water are tough to get down. But he tries anyway.

"It will take me a year to grow back in to my clothes...I'll have to finish the school year in baggy bell bottoms," Keen says referring to his 1970's striped bell bottoms that he actually wore to Henry Clay High School (HCHS) in the 1970's and brings to class when his students study this era. Why he kept that particular pair of pants remains a mystery. So the thought of Dr. Babbage wearing those jeans to class makes us both laugh—well I laugh and Keen makes that face that says, "Why is that funny?" Uh huh.

The feeding tube is behaving now and Keen has almost reached his goal of fluid per hour. The staff will work to get him off the pump so he can take the liquid food in shorter periods of time and go about his life. We have been talking about all the yummy things we can put through that tube. Gratefully he won't be able to taste any of it!

Although Keen isn't ready to start training for a 10K we talk about running one this summer. It is so good to have plans that take us beyond this hospital and this diagnosis.

We remain grateful for you and for the notes, thoughts, and especially the prayers. Keen says pray, pray more, keep praying...we want a miracle as big as the Easter resurrection—and we want it for everyone who is suffering right now.

# Wednesday, Dec 8, 2010

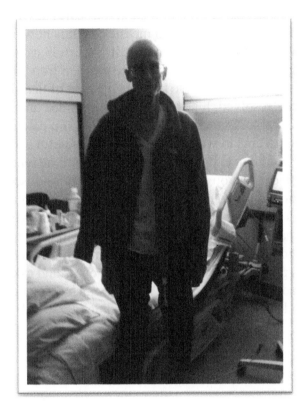

    With his arm around my shoulder, all six feet three inches of Keen walked today, in his sweatpants and fleece jacket, around the perimeter of the third floor of Markey Cancer Center. Nurses and techs came out of patient rooms to see who the "celebrity" was when they heard colleagues saying, "Well look who it is" and "I had no idea you were that tall!" The doctors who had gathered at the nurses' station took a break from their conversation to smile and encourage Keen on his walk-about the floor. It was a sight to behold.

    Keen's IV fluid has been discontinued except for an occasional boost of potassium and he is "eating" well through his feeding tube. Radiation has continued, with only five treatments remaining. Keen plans to leave the hospital on Friday morning—if all goes well. It was a day of smiles and prayers of gratitude.

"I think I could be cast as a villain in Hollywood movie," Keen said as he looked at himself in the mirror. We laughed and began to imagine how *that* story might be told. Keen has lost a lot of weight, but he has decided not to look at the scales anymore. Scales only tell part of the story. The real measurement is how Keen feels. He has color in his face, "What color is it?" Keen likes to ask, and he is moving again. Although his ankles are swollen from all the IV fluid, a few days up and mobile should take care of that. His pneumonia has resolved, his colon bug has subsided and his pain level is manageable. In fact, he is only using a pain patch at this point, and that seems to work. So much to be grateful about.

Keen will come "home" to our house until he ready to move back to his place. As you might imagine life at our house is a bit different than the one Keen has known for the past 30-plus years...things don't usually work as smoothly here. So Keen, always the teacher, has helped us find new "strategies" to keep up with lost and misplaced items like car keys, cell phones and wallets. I told Keen what a positive influence he has been on us and asked if any of our habits had rubbed off on him. Without much delay he looked pensively and said, "I bought new jeans, didn't I?" Ugh!

# Life Lesson: Each Day Matters

I had one day between the cancer diagnosis on Tuesday, October 12 and the start of treatments on Thursday, October 14. Most of Wednesday, October 13 was spent at the high school where I was a teacher. I had to painfully, tearfully and honestly tell my students that I would be gone for several months. I had to make plans with the school administrators and some teaching colleagues for my classes. I also had to see two doctors to prepare for treatments.

October 13 was also a day to visit my mother in her hospital room. The surgery she had recently did reveal abdominal cancer, but no treatment options were seriously considered. With her very fragile and declining health, cancer treatments would have been cruel. Instead, she was placed in Hospice care so her final days could be peaceful and painless.

I was very thankful that my mother did not have to be told that I had cancer. My brother and sister-in-law were with me when I was given the cancer diagnosis. On Wednesday, October 13, at the hospital where my mother was a patient, I spoke with my niece and nephews to tell them that I had cancer. They were watching their grandmother die. Now they were hearing news which meant their uncle could die. These were very difficult days.

It became obvious very quickly to me that a decision was necessary. The fact in October 2010 was that Keen has cancer. The decision was whether or not cancer had Keen.

What does that mean? It means I had to decide in my mind, heart and soul whether being a cancer patient would define me or whether I would define what it meant to be a cancer patient. I chose to take control over what I could still control.

I would visit my mother. I would pray with her and for her. I would keep talking to her even after she could not respond. I would express love to my mother then and love for my mother always. Cancer could not prevent that.

I would make all necessary arrangements for my students. Their education would not be interrupted while my career was interrupted. Students, colleagues and I would find ways to keep in touch by mail, email and visits.

I had cancer, but cancer did not have me. Cancer did not have me in its grips. Cancer did not have control of my thoughts, my beliefs, my hopes, my determination, my willingness to fight back or my faith.

I was still me. Cancer would require that some characteristics of mine become more defined and more certain. Some people tell me that they are amazed at the courage that teachers have to enter the classroom daily. Contrasting 35 days in the classroom with 35 days going into the radiation treatment machine says the courage required to endure the harsh, brutal, exhausting radiation process far surpasses the abundant courage needed to teach.

Cancer would challenge me to find a new depth of courage, of determination, of resilience, of faith, of resolve, of persistence, of hope and of confidence.

I had cancer. I had to deal with the life-threatening reality of cancer. But cancer did not have me. Cancer had to deal with my life affirming resources of medical science, Christian faith, devoted family, caring students, loyal friends and the human virtues including a stubborn determination to endure some of the worst conditions a human can face to develop and display some of the best qualities a human can acquire.

I had cancer. Cancer did not have me, except as a fully determined opponent. How long I would live was unknown. How honorably and persistently would I affirm life whatever the length of time given to me? Completely.

The cancer patient has cancer. Cancer acts to have the cancer patient, meaning cancer acts to possess, own and destroy the patient. By fighting back honorably, confidently, persistently, completely, the cancer patient adds to the nobility, the goodness, the honor, the integrity, the virtue, the example within his or her life and inspires such fullness of living in others.

I had cancer. I took that personally. I wanted cancer to regret being in my body and being in my life. Who would win? I declared victory from the start. Fighting back was victorious. Getting treatments was victorious. Asking people to pray for me was victorious. Building a vast support network of family and friends was victorious.

The evil of cancer would be surpassed by the applied goodness of caring people. Cancer has no match for that. I had cancer, but cancer did not have and would never have my thoughts, my attitude, my convictions, my beliefs, my family, my friends, my faith or my depth of determination.

It was not guaranteed that I would get well. I decided to guarantee that I would fight back very well. I had cancer. Cancer did not have me. Cancer would not have me.

I thought often of what my dear mother had told us days before her death, "If I die, do not grieve. Rejoice that I lived a good life."

My version of that became, "If I die do not grieve. Rejoice that I fought the good fight."

I was in a war. Wars have fatalities, wounds, survivors. Would I die, be wounded or survive? That was to be determined. I could determine what type of soldier I would be in this war, now and forever.

\*　　　\*　　　\*

In addition to feeling awful, in addition to being dehydrated, in addition to losing 20% of my body weight, in addition to being hospitalized for 10 days, in addition to receiving chemotherapy and radiation treatments, it was obvious that I was very, very sick because I could not go to work.

In the 17 years with my current employer, I had missed 12 days prior to the cancer diagnosis. I was away from work for 10 days in 1996 to recover from ulcer surgery. I was away from work for two additional days when my mother had two surgeries. Now, I was in the midst of missing months of work.

If missing work communicated to me that I was very severely sick, the solution was to return to work. In October, November and December 2010, such a return was impossible. In January, after the radiation treatments had been completed the prior month, after the January round of chemotherapy was finished, I was given permission to return to work for one hour on one day. Rejoice and give thanks.

Most of my career has been in education. When I was diagnosed with cancer I was in my 27$^{th}$ year as either a teacher or a school administrator. In October 2010, I was teaching United States History and Political Science to high school students. On one day in late January 2011, I went to school and taught one class just to see if I could still do that work.

Chemotherapy and radiation treatments had so effectively overpowered the cancer that in February I would be told that there were no signs of cancer. Rejoice. Shed tears. Give thanks.

Teaching therapy, given to me for one hour on one day in January 2011, nourished my body, nurtured my soul, invigorated my heart and energized my mind. Cancer had attacked my body and had imposed serious damage. But I could still teach. One of the biggest parts of my life—my job, my occupation, my vocation, my career—could still function.

One hour of work on one day did not equal full recovery and did not mean an instant return to full-time work could begin. What did that one hour mean?

It meant that for one hour cancer had been completely defeated.

The students in my Political Science class were very supportive on that January day. They looked past my dreadful appearance—I weighed 140 pounds, down from 175, and at six feet three inches tall, 140 pounds barely covers a body. My hair was gone, a casualty of chemotherapy. But we could discuss and analyze Political Science in January as we had in October.

Being back at work for one hour was pure joy. It was a way to tell myself that the worst of this cancer war was over. It was a way to declare one victory.

It is difficult, perhaps impossible, for a cancer patient to obtain 100% victory over cancer. Even if the cancer is completely removed by surgery and/or treatment, the body has been through and remains in a war. There will be many battle scars that never fade.

Whenever possible, a cancer patient needs to create victories. During the months or years of treatment, it is helpful to find beneficial parts of life which can be maintained exactly or nearly as they were before cancer appeared. If you always went to church keep going to church if that is medically allowed. If it is not allowed for you to be out in a group, have church come to you. Church services can be listened to on the radio or watched on television. A few church members can join you for a small community worship service at your home.

If you were a great cook before cancer arrived, keep cooking. The food may not appeal to you. A feeding tube may be the way you get nourishment. But cooking has value and meaning for you, so cook. Share the food with family and friends.

If you were accustomed to getting much exercise before cancer, it may be quite difficult to do much physical activity during cancer treatments or soon after cancer treatments. Create small victories. When I was hospitalized, I was bedridden. After five or six days, my family encouraged me to try walking in the hospital hallway. With their encouragement, a very short walk was completed. The hospital staff cheered. It was not the eight miles I used to run, but it was more than being bedridden had included. A small victory, but a victory.

When you are at war with cancer, cancer keeps score. Cancer counts the days you miss work as points in the cancer column. Cancer counts your loss of hair, your loss of weight, your loss of appetite, your new aches and pains, your moments of doubt and despair, your sickness itself as points in the cancer column.

Part of fighting back is to create fights that you win. Hold onto as many good parts of life as possible despite the cancer war you are in. Think of a promise you made yourself years ago and create the plan which begins to make that promise come true. Create victories. Be victorious. Win every time you can. Create situations that can become victories.

Cancer acts to kill you. If it cannot kill you, cancer acts to destroy you, to devastate you, to make you despair about being alive, to wreck your life.

Amid the genuine awfulness which cancer is and which cancer wickedly injects into your life, you can counter punch cancer with victories that you inject into your life while you are fighting cancer. Make many small victories a significant part of the big war you wage against cancer.

*     *     *

There are phases in the war against cancer. The number of phases and the exact content of each phase will vary from person to person. The initial phase is fairly similar for all cancer patients. This first phase begins with a medical doctor stating that you have cancer. Exactly what the physician says will vary from doctor to doctor, but the message is clear, certain, painful, frightening, disappointing, awful and abrupt.

No person is ever fully prepared to be told "you have cancer." I could see the edge of my cancerous sinus tumor in my left nostril, but I could not diagnose it. After a Friday, October 1, 2010 CT scan and a Monday, October 4, 2010 MRI, the expectation grew that this could be and likely was cancer.

Even when the words "you have cancer" come with little or no surprise, they come with the force of a casket being dropped on you. Phase one is the official diagnosis, but there is more to phase one. "Will I die?" "Can this be treated?" "Will the treatments work?" "Will the treatments make me sick?" "What chance do I have of living through this?" "While I get treatments, can I still go to work?"

In my case, phase one included all of those questions and many more. I spent eight hours with doctors and their colleagues on the day I was diagnosed. A PET scan was needed that day to see if the cancer was localized in the sinus area or if it had spread. The word metastasize became a major emphasis. The good news was that the cancer was in and near the sinus area only.

It may seem to be unusual thinking and peculiar thinking to say it is good news to have cancer in only one area, but once you have cancer you search for the slightest sliver of encouraging news.

Time was spent with an oncologist including being shown a picture of my face, skull and brain areas. The tumor was massive. The tumor was dangerously close to the left optic nerve. The tumor had begun penetrating the brain. The war against cancer had begun. Cancer had attacked first. The day of diagnosis, Tuesday, October 12, 2010 became "a date which will live in infamy" to borrow Franklin Roosevelt's words from his December 8, 1941 declaration of war speech.

The difference? World War II came to an end in August 1945. The war a cancer patient wages against cancer has no such ending. The war endures throughout your remaining days, weeks, months, years or decades. There are wounds, injuries, casualties, deaths, atrocities, heroics, valor, honor, courage, attacks and counter attacks in war, including the war against cancer.

Treatments begin and the war is taken to cancer. A tumor or tumors may shrink. Cancer cells may be destroyed. Side effects emerge. You feel worse before you feel better, if you feel better.

Getting rid of cancer is essential, but your body may have new difficulties which are the result of cancer treatments. Getting rid of cancer is a vital victory, but it is not a total victory or a permanent victory. Cancer can return. Side effects can last five years, 10 years, forever. Side effects can worsen. New side effects can appear on a cruel time-released schedule.

Fighting cancer is total war which takes your total effort until remission is established. Then fighting cancer includes frequent monitoring, frequent tests, new concerns about any health condition that happens—is this related to cancer or to cancer treatment or to new cancer? Life is never what it was once the war with cancer begins. Never.

If the war is lost and the cancer patient dies, there is much sorrow, many tears and deep regret. For friends and family of a cancer patient who died, the war against cancer remains. Cancer continues to cause heart break for survivors.

Each day matters. Each moment matters. We measure life in years. A 20th reunion. A 16th birthday. 30 years living in the same home. Yet, we live life in moments.

The moments a couple says "I do" and then the pastor says "I now pronounce you husband and wife." The moment a child is born. The moment a college graduate is handed a diploma. The moment a 75-year-old blows out birthday candles on a cake, with help from grandchildren.

Cancer patients learn to appreciate each moment and to live in this moment, right here, right now.

# Moving Home

Caregivers do not always take care of themselves. It can be a vicious cycle of caring for a sick loved one and wanting to be needed, while setting necessary boundaries and practicing good self-care. Keen had moved into our home before Thanksgiving. While he was taking high doses of pain medicine we decided Keen needed more support, so he came to stay with us. It was not a big discussion; rather it was more a matter of fact conclusion. This new arrangement simplified transportation to and from his treatment and added a dimension of support that Keen would not have living alone in his home. It all made perfect sense, and besides, I *had* promised Nana.

So when our annual Thanksgiving trip to Florida was discussed it seemed a foregone conclusion that I would stay home and care for Keen while the family traveled to Florida for a much needed break. I was adamant about the family making the trip. There was very little discussion about it which was, in hindsight, our first mistake. And so I helped pack up my family for the trip and took them to the airport. It was only then that the stark reality hit me; I was going to be home by myself with Keen, without the rest of my family and with no plans to celebrate Thanksgiving.

I was miserable. Looking back on that decision it seems almost comical that I thought everyone else needed a break except the caregiver herself. It was a mistake. Holidays can be difficult under the best of circumstances. Caregivers must be brutally honest about what they can and cannot sacrifice for the person for whom they are caring. And in this case, Keen was my *husband's* brother. Maybe I had taken on more than was expected for a sister-in-law.

My spiritual director (a trained, experienced, wise and holy person who guides and helps an individual deepen his or her relationship with the Divine through a process of reflection and prayer) helped me to look more closely at this decision and make a better one when a larger decision about intensive home care needed to be made—around the clock care for Keen after he was discharged from the hospital. Of course, he would come home with us and we would take care of him. She sat me down and would not hear of me leaving the room until I had come up with another option. One that provided an alternative to turning our home into a makeshift hospital with around the clock care provided by our family. She was determined to help me find options that would relieve me of full-time care giving responsibilities over the Christmas holiday and provide a home where our children could rest during their school breaks. She helped me to see that enacting my original plan could potentially harm Keen's recovery, not to mention what it would mean to our family.

I made some phone calls and was able to put into action a plan that would enable Keen to stay at his own home after he was discharged from the hospital while providing the care he needed to recuperate. It was a win-win.

The way you know that a decision is a good one is how you feel afterwards. My breathing had slowed down, and my heart felt lighter. There was a peacefulness about the decision that I had not expected to feel. It was immediate. My spiritual director, Sr. Frances, saw it on my face and I saw that knowing smile appear on hers.

Looking back over the time spent in giving care, this was the single best decision made. It kept me positive and prevented me from becoming resentful and angry. Caregivers need help sorting out their thoughts and feelings, especially when difficult decisions need to be made. Seeking guidance from wise friends and professionals can help keep peace in families and the hearts of caregivers.

# Friday, Dec 10, 2010

Keen is all packed up and ready to leave Markey, ending a "23 hour" stay that began last Tuesday. It has been quite a journey—and I don't think he is sad to be saying goodbye to the staff, even though they have been exceptional. We have around the clock care planned for Keen until he is feeling stronger and steadier. He wrote last night to say "I just finished supper: two cans of yummy Jevity tube feeding nutrition." We have much to celebrate on this near balmy Friday afternoon!

# Tuesday, Dec 14, 2010

Keen finished his 33rd of 35 radiation treatments this morning. They only get more difficult. Keen's prayers are more serious these days, and he prays with more urgency. It is as if I can hear his mother finish the prayer for him with an emphatic "Amen" and then upon reflection adding, "PLEASE, Amen."

Keen walks more slowly. He can imagine the day when he releases the "hold" button on life and starts living again. On THAT day as the Advent readings speak so clearly about, there will be great rejoicing in heaven and on earth.

When asked what he looks forward to most Keen answers, "Being back in the classroom with my students and tasting food again." It sounds so simple.

Keen's home has been a place of healing and peace. He has 24 hour care 7 days a week. That will continue for a couple of weeks, until the cumulative effects of radiation subside and he gains strength and confidence. Friends visit regularly and Keen keeps in touch using his iPhone. He has become a fan of "texting." For a man who could never find a good reason to carry a cell phone, he has mastered his iPhone.

A group of Christmas carolers, students and adults from church, serenaded Keen on Sunday. His gratitude was expressed through tears of joy.

In about four weeks Keen should begin feeling more like himself. "It can't happen soon enough," Keen says. In mid-January, Keen will have another MRI to determine if further treatment is necessary. We are hopeful that the radiation and Chemotherapy along with massive doses of prayer will knock out the cancer, but if not there are other options for treatment.

# Thursday, Dec 16, 2010

We are celebrating! Today Keen completed 35 of 35 radiation treatments. It has been a rugged seven weeks, with many obstacles along the way, but this morning we were high fiving and all smiles. Even the obturator went in without an issue—no gagging, nothing. Yesterday Keen decided to think of it as a candy bar. When I asked him to name his favorite childhood candy bar he responded after just a moment's thought and said, "Zagnut, Snickers and PayDay." Soon and very soon, he will eat his first candy bar post-radiation and actually taste it. It is a day we long for.

Although the radiation doctor cautioned us that Christmas week could be his hardest week (Keen still wonders how it gets harder), after that he should begin the healing process. Swallowing will come back gradually and the mouth and throat will begin healing. He will start feeling better the week after Christmas, according to his doctor, just in time to begin his 4th round of Chemotherapy which happens Dec 28 to 30. Sometime in mid January another MRI will be taken to determine what comes next.

# Life Lesson: To Every Problem There is an Equal and Opposite Plan of Attack

Cancer is physical. Cancer attacks the body. Cancer declares war on your body. There is no reason for cancer to be allowed to attack your thoughts, your ability to hope, your beliefs, your mind, your heart, your soul.

Cancer is physical. Human beings are physical, but we are much more. We can love, care, believe, hope, dream, plan and think. Cancer can do none of that.

Cancer fights us physically. Part of our fighting back against cancer is physical. Chemotherapy goes into the body and physically confronts cancer. Radiation is sent into the body and confronts cancer. The physical invasion and the physical attack of cancer must be countered by a stronger, relentless, precise physical counter attack.

The other weapons which are in the human arsenal must be applied in the war against cancer.

Think, but not of fantasies or of magic. Think about what caused the cancer. Ask the doctors what caused the cancer. Analyze your life to identify any cancer causing habits, practices, actions. Eliminate all of those habits, practices, actions now and forever.

My analysis and thinking began by asking one Ear, Nose and Throat doctor what caused the cancer. I was ready and willing to stop any cancer-causing actions in my life. I was ready and willing to start any cancer-fighting actions in my life.

The answer was, "It is nothing that you did and nothing that you did not do. It is just out of control cells."

My thinking then turned to how can I increase the effectiveness of the treatment I would receive? I could accept them willingly, optimistically, thankfully and cooperatively. I could not think the chemotherapy into working better or harder. I could think about chemotherapy in ways that made the many hours of that therapy create learning.

It was important for me to fully understand what was being done to me, how it was being done, why it was being done in this way and what options there were, if any.

It was also very important that my cancer war be educational for medical science. Cancer cannot learn about itself, but human beings can learn about cancer from the experience of each patient. Sinus cancer is very rare so my experience could provide insights and knowledge for doctors, medical students and other healthcare professionals.

My eagerness to learn and my eagerness for the medical profession to learn from my cancer war were ways to show cancer that it was up against an army which would fight now and forever. This is a war to the last cancer cell. This is also a war against cancer, one would hope, to help end all wars against cancer, to borrow a thought from Woodrow Wilson about World War I being the war to end all wars.

Wilson's plan did not work. My thought about using my war with cancer to help identify weapons which will help win the ultimate, complete, total war with cancer, I hope will have better results.

As the war with cancer continues, I increasingly work to reduce the impact the war has on me. Cancer will not change my beliefs, so I continue to pray, to read the Bible, to attend church. Cancer will not change my dreams, so I continue to envision and work toward my ideal job. Cancer will not change my commitments, so I continue to honor and to cherish my family responsibilities.

Cancer has reduced my strength, my weight and my athletic endurance. For now. I cannot yet exercise as I did before cancer; however, when I do minimal exercise it is with maximum delight. As I exercise, I am thankful for what I can do. Anything above nothing is another defeat of cancer's lingering efforts. What exercise I can get now is another way of saying, "Take that cancer."

Cancer wants us to think that life has become evil and is picking on cancer patients. Life is not evil. Cancer is evil. Cancer cannot be allowed to control our thoughts about life itself.

This brings up the question of "why me?" which a cancer patient might be inclined to ask. The question is understandable, but may not be very productive. For a person who has smoked tobacco products, getting cancer could be due to smoking those products. The answer to "why me" is because you smoked tobacco products.

Another person who never smoked tobacco products and who never did any action known to be cancer-causing could still have cancer. Why did cancer happen to that person? The benefit of asking the "why me" question is to objectively evaluate your life so all possible cancer-causing action can be removed. The "why me" question is otherwise unproductive if all it does is consume mental energy and create new anguish.

The "why" of "why me" may never be known. The me of "why me" is known. Cancer is at war with me. Cancer is at war with you. The larger question is how, not why. The how question is "How will I fight back?" You did not decide to have cancer. You do get to decide how you will fight cancer. Even with cancer, the human has advantages. The human mind, heart and soul are outside of cancer's reach if we do not let cancer touch them. Hold onto your mind, heart and soul. Use them in the war against cancer. Cancer has no equivalent tactic to match the human mind, heart and soul.

One additional thought. In books I have written about teaching and about school administration, I have often expressed the confident conclusion that "To every problem there is an equal and opposite solution." That statement is true about education. When the right decisions are made and the right actions are taken plus when the wrong decisions are not made and when the wrong actions are avoided, any educational problem can be solved.

That is not true with cancer. There are some cancer problems for which a solution does not exist. Some cancer patients are told, "It is too late. The disease is too far along. We are so sorry, but no treatment would help. No surgery would help." Some cancer patients are told, "The cancer is resisting the treatments. There is nothing else we can try."

Cancer can be treated successfully only to return later. Cancer can be treated effectively only for the patient to have lifelong limitations due to side effects of and collateral damage from the treatments. The return of cancer cannot be fully prevented. The side effects and collateral damage cannot be avoided and cannot always be corrected.

For some problems related to cancer there is no solution;

however, there is always a plan of attack. What is the plan of attack when a cancer patient is told that nothing can be done and that life will end in six months? With the strength you have, make the most of those six months. See your loved ones as often as possible. Write letters to family members and to friends expressing the deepest thoughts. Prepare your funeral. Update your will. Pray for a miracle. Get a second opinion. Make every moment count. Do what matters most. Waste no time. To the extent that your health allows, put the most into and get the most out of each day.

*  *  *

To every problem there is an equal and opposite plan of attack. In the treatment of cancer, machines and other sophisticated technological equipment are often used as parts of the plan of attack. The CT scan and MRI machines are highly complex devices which provide a close look into the body. Doctors can use the images from these machines to help diagnose, to monitor progress and to fine tune treatment.

While these machines can measure and depict the body, the cancer patient has an opportunity to measure his or her heart, mind and soul. As the cancer patient fine tunes his or her heart, mind and soul the war against cancer gains new strength, more powerful weapons and a foundation of resolve that will not break.

My body was given 35 doses of radiation treatment. I was initially told that after two or three weeks of treatments, there would be physical difficulties. The schedule was to have treatments five days per week for seven weeks. Easy, I thought, all I do is show up, lie down on the table, get moved into the radiation machine tunnel, stay absolutely motionless for seven minutes, exit the tunnel and go home.

I was told that the computers ran for over a week to perfectly plan the attack against the cancer in my sinus area. While that was being done, one day I was fitted with an upper body cage which the technicians called a mask. The device resembles a chain link fence design. It goes from your chest to your head and is placed over you each day. Then it is snapped into place which means that the patient is restrained onto the table which will then slide into the radiation machine tunnel. You must not move and, for the upper body, you cannot move. The Bible verse from Psalm 46:10 applies quite practically: "Be still and know that I am God."

For the first and second days of radiation treatment, I was quite intrigued with the machine, the sounds, the process and the procedure. The very capable technicians answered all of my questions. I was determined to arrive at the radiation center each day with energy, hope, optimism and joy. The technicians work with some very sick people and I wanted to brighten the atmosphere for everyone.

My enthusiastic plan of attack worked well for 11 days. On day 12, I could barely walk into the radiation room. I needed help getting onto the table. It was increasingly difficult to force the large mouth piece beyond my lips, but it had to be done so the collateral damage to the tongue and mouth could be reduced.

Day 12 was awful, discouraging, agonizing and filled with doubt. The accumulated impact of radiation and chemotherapy was shrinking the tumor. The daily measures showed certain progress. The accumulated impact of radiation and chemotherapy had nearly depleted me of energy, appetite, the ability to swallow and any ability to bring joy, optimism and energy into the radiation room. The war had become increasingly intense.

I had to endure. I must persist. The only option was to endure. How? Day 13 would be worse. Day 14 would be worse than that. The disease of cancer can be deadly. I knew that. Must the treatments make the cancer patient feel closer to death than the disease alone makes you feel? Certainly there is a plan of attack to confront this new Day 12 of radiation problem.

I am a Christian. The search for a plan of attack was successful right in the radiation room. While lying on the table, head-locked in place, prior to being moved into the radiation tunnel, my only way to look was straight up. In the ceiling above the table was a tile that had a portion cut out. There was a camera or other monitoring machinery in the ceiling looking down at the table and the patient. That cut out portion was in the shape of a cross. For a Christian that was a reminder to, as 2 Timothy 4:7 tell us "Fight the good fight. Keep the faith. Finish the race."

Day 12 was trench warfare. Cancer's war against me had

become more brutal, more vicious, more agonizing, more demanding, more aggressive and more potent. Cancer was using conventional warfare, guerilla warfare and atomic warfare simultaneously. Cancer's plan of attack was now obvious—total war. What would my counter plan of attack be?

When a person intends to make progress with weightlifting, the workout has to change often. If an exercise routine includes use of 50-pound weights for one specific movement, the body will get accustomed to lifting 50 pounds. Progress will require a new challenge, a new demand on the muscles. 55 pounds must be attempted to force the development of new muscular strength.

Cancer was hitting me with stronger weapons. I had to dig deeper to fight back. Going from 50 pounds to 55 pounds requires extra effort from the athlete. Going from the tranquility of day 11 in the radiation room to the difficulty of day 12 would require more effort; each following day would be equivalent to the weightlifter adding more weight to a workout.

Could I lift 55 pounds today in the war against cancer? Could I lift 60 pounds tomorrow? I had to. There was no choice. No option. No alternative. It had to be done, and I had to do it.

The weightlifter uses more than muscle and physical force to lift weights. Where does the desire, the effort, the push, the never give up determination of the weightlifter originate? In the human will to achieve. In the human heart to excel. In the human mind to push. In the soul of a person who finds power in belief that propels tangible results in the physical realm.

My revised plan of attack was, in a word, more. Attack. Attack more. Keep attacking.

# Monday, December 20, 2010

This is a difficult week on many levels. The accumulated effects of radiation create new physical problems including weariness and sleeplessness. Although the tube feedings are going well, they also create new problems in the GI tract. For every treatment there is a consequence it seems. However the physical side effects do not begin to take into account the pervasive sense of loss of day to day "living." There is no way to quantify how Keen feels about the loss of time in the classroom with his students and the day-to-day endorphin surge surrounding life at Henry Clay High School. While life goes on all around him, Keen remains in an oppressive holding pattern that is magnified during the Christmas season.

This is a good time to send CaringBridge notes, text messages, cards and encouraging thoughts. After his appointment with his cancer doctor today he said, "I just wish everyone would stop saying 'It's ok.' It's NOT ok," he said with as much emphasis as he could muster. That's when I got right in his face and reminded him that this is exactly what the radiation doctors predicted would be his worst week post-radiation and it will simply take time to feel like himself again. Healing will begin next week. He will get that week to recover some before his fourth round of chemo Jan 4 to 6.

So, that's where we are today. Thanks for the ways in which you have ministered to Keen throughout the course of this diagnosis and treatment. Unfortunately, there are no shortcuts and there is no way around the suffering.

# Wednesday, December 22, 2010

I was so thrilled to get this text today from the night helper that I wanted to share it with you. Keen and I are at the ENT doctor this morning. The doctor is working to get some of the accumulated "wallpaper paste" out of his nose so he can breathe again. The scorched throat will begin healing soon which will make swallowing a more reasonable request. The cumulative effects of radiation to the eyes, nose, throat and ears (any orifice that can get clogged, will) are treacherous. Keen just said to the doctor who helped get some of the gunk out of his nose, "I can already tell a difference," to which the doctor responded, "It will come back." Ah a momentary victory—we will take it!

From the helper:

"Everything is wonderful such a improvement more vigor alert very talkative slept from 11 to about 4am ... nose mouth and eye care"

"right bk to sleep and snored till i had to wake him 4 shower hes n a great frame of mind faith love and all those wonderful prayers packed a punch"

# Wednesday, Dec 29, 2010

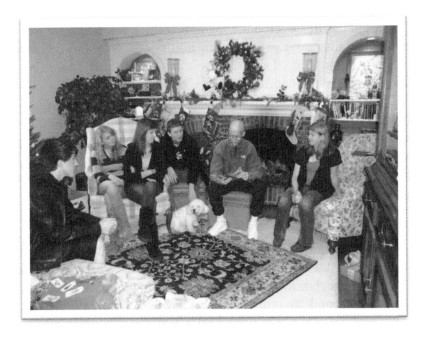

There is nothing like a gathering of students to lift your spirits. Today Keen visited with a group of his students and enjoyed every second of the time together. "What does it mean that we just had elections and Congress is passing bills like crazy?" Dr. Babbage asked his students. "They are trying to get as much passed as possible before the new candidates take office," Margaret correctly answered. Dr. Babbage clapped his hands.

The side effects from radiation are beginning to ease. The 24/7 home care has ended and Keen is finding some sense of rhythm to his days. "It helps to have things to look forward to," Keen confided in the car today. Yes, the days at home can get long and lonely without text messages from friends and family, phone calls, visits and planned activities. So we make plans.

Today, Keen will work on swallowing some jello. He associates swallowing food with all things bad, so the barrier to swallowing becomes more than a physical impediment. But this too shall pass. We remind ourselves often of the temporariness of the multiple side effects of 35 radiation treatments and three rounds of chemo (soon to be four). So the doctors were right when they said, Christmas will be your hardest week, but New Years will be better. Check.

Keen has discovered the joy of a warm neck scarf. He demonstrated his new scarf wrapping ability on Christmas day when his nephew Brian said, "I don't know how to tie a scarf." Keen's response was, "Watch and learn."

On Christmas Day we read aloud Jesse Stuart's short story "Santa's Visit" that was published in the *Lexington Herald Leader* on Christmas Eve. It was moving and motivational and reminded us of our many blessings. We read it again today as we gathered in a circle around the living room with each student taking a turn to read aloud a few paragraphs. It was one those "wholesome, G-rated" activities that Keen encourages, invites and welcomes in his classroom.

We are continually amazed by Keen's students and the gentle ways they minister to him. Keen looks forward to the day when he can return to his classroom, where he will enjoy preparing lessons for his students and the ordinariness of living day-by-day. We are learning that life is never the same after a cancer diagnosis. Adjusting to a "new normal" presents its own daily learning curve. And so we learn and adjust and move on. We remain grateful for all the ways you walk this journey with us. Happy New Year!

# Life Lesson: There is Much to be Thankful For

Some days I struggle. Some days I struggle more. There are no struggle-free days.

Some days I feel bad. Other days I feel worse. I never feel good.

Yet, there is much to be thankful for.

Some days the side effects cause problems. Some days the side effects cause severe problems. The side effects are always there. They are permanent. They have not improved. They have worsened.

Still there is much to be thankful for.

I used to exercise vigorously. I used to run many miles often. I used to have endless energy. None of that happens now.

I used to age one year at a time. Cancer and cancer treatments accelerated the aging process. My body is much older than my birth certificate indicates.

I can go to work. I can walk the dog. I can read. I can think. I can pray. I can remember. I can talk. The I cans outnumber the I cannots. The I cans are more important than the I cannots.

There is much to be thankful for.

At the worst moments of the most intense parts of the forever war with cancer, there has been agony, there has been despair, there was a limit that was reached. Then a new "limit" was set and that was not reached because it is infinite.

There is much to question, much to analyze, much to evaluate, much to endure, much to suffer, much to lose, much to cry about and much to be apprehensive about. All of that is real. All of that is encountered. All of that need not be overpowering.

Even during the forever war with cancer, there is much to be thankful for. I choose to be thankful. Take that, cancer.

*     *     *

A cancer patient could be asked this kind of question: "Do you think it is unfair that you have cancer? Is life picking on you?

Why didn't God keep this from happening to you?"

My responses to that frame of mind are from a different perspective.

I was born into a wonderful family. My dear parents were devoted to my brother and me. We were given so many good childhood and teenage experiences. We were taught so well. We were reared so well.

I knew my mother's parents quite well. We visited them every week or two. They were the most loving grandparents a child could have. When our family had some difficulties, they were the solid rock foundation which kept everything together. Their integrity, honor, virtue, wisdom, faith, love, goodness and example are what I continue to find guidance from. I am thankful.

I was able to earn a doctorate from the University of Kentucky. I have been able to write 16 published books about education. I have had meaningful experiences in 29 years as an educator.

As a 22-year-old college senior I was hired by the Procter & Gamble Company to work in advertising. I had four years of vital experiences at that company which is among the world's best in many ways. My colleagues there set standards for work ethic, teamwork, integrity, management, leadership, budgeting, communication and listening to consumers, which have shaped my career and my life.

In 1980, I was given the pure joy of walking 430 miles from St. Louis, Missouri to Cincinnati, Ohio as I carried the opening day baseball. I gave the ball to the March of Dimes poster child who threw it to a Cincinnati Reds' player to start the season.

I have the dearest relatives. My brother, sister-in-law, nephews, niece and their dog are treasured and cherished by me. There is much to be thankful for.

Amid all of those blessings in life, how can I condemn life because I am in a forever war with cancer? Do I make the most of life or do I curse life for the evil of cancer? I choose to make the most of life. Why let cancer have any edge? Why let the evil of cancer cancel out the abundant goodness of many other parts of life?

Is it unfair that I have had cancer? Wrong question. Is it unfair to let cancer cancel the vast goodness in life? Yes, so one way to beat cancer is to never let it negate prior, current and hoped for future goodness.

*     *     *

I have to wear hearing aids for the rest of my life because the type of chemotherapy I had damaged my hearing.

I wake up during each night because my mouth and my throat are so dry it hurts. Radiation treatments damaged my saliva system.

I mop my eyes throughout the day because radiation treatments destroyed the tear ducts. I have minimal breathing and sometimes no breathing through my left nostril due to the tumor and the radiation treatments.

Each morning when I wake up it takes about two to five minutes to get my eyes to open. A washcloth with warm water usually has to be applied. This is another side effect of radiation.

I am sleepy at 7:30 p.m. and often in bed by 8:00 p.m. That is a post-cancer schedule.

Before cancer I ran 20 to 25 miles weekly. My after cancer body has not allowed any miles of running.

There is much to be thankful for.

I lost 35 pounds during the months of cancer treatment. I was already thin. 15 pounds have been gained back in over two years.

My taste buds do not work. They were radiated. I pick up a tiny taste from some foods and no taste from others.

I have needed two surgeries since the cancer treatments ended. Two more surgeries are needed soon. All of these are due to cancer treatment side effects.

I spend a lot of time with doctors. I have regularly scheduled CT scans and MRI tests.

I never feel as energetic as I did before cancer.

I never feel good. My best days are when I feel less bad than on my usual days. On my worst days, I long for a usual day of feeling just bad instead of feeling awful.

Because part of the tumor was in my brain, radiation impacted part of my brain. Occasionally I am a second slow when remembering a fact or a name.

I am told that the radiation also impacted the part of the brain that governs social interaction. I am less inclined to be outgoing than I was before cancer.

I once had a large, expanding, aggressive, cancerous tumor in my sinus area, near my eyes and entering my brain. I have been cancer free for over two years.

There is much to be thankful for.

*     *     *

On Tuesday, April 9, 2013, there is much to be thankful for. I have survived for two and a half years since being told that there was a large, aggressive cancerous tumor in my sinus area, entering my brain and posing a serious threat to the left optic nerve. There were many days in October, November and December 2010 when survival was in doubt and, to be blunt, was unlikely.

Yet, the perspective that there is much to be thankful for does not deny the reality of problems; rather, it makes the most of what is good while still honestly addressing what is difficult, serious and deadly.

When asked how I feel or how I am doing my answer continues to be "There is much to be thankful for" because this is true and because that attitude gives me an edge. I need that edge.

On Tuesday, April 9, 2013 there is much to be concerned about. I spent three and a half hours yesterday at a medical facility. There are problems with my left optic nerve. It is swollen. The best judgment now is that there was a "stroke" meaning that a blood vessel which should deliver nourishing blood to that optic nerve failed to do so. My vision is still functional. I can see. There is much to be thankful for. I have some minimal visual distortions with my left eye. There is much to be concerned about.

What has caused this new problem with the left optic nerve? How long has the problem been developing? What will happen next? Is there any treatment? Such questions can consume your time, thoughts, energy and more. I am asking those questions. We will get answers. But I am going to work today. I got exercise early this morning. I will attend a book signing event tonight. Life does go on.

But there is much to be concerned about. Has cancer

returned? Is a new tumor or are new tumors causing the optic nerve problem? Within two weeks, I may have had a lumbar puncture more commonly known as a spinal tap. That will help identify whether cancer may be present. If those test results are abnormal, there will be more tests about cancer. If cancer is present again, well, there will be a plan of attack. Faith, family, friends will team up anew; medical science will mount an assault.

If those results are normal, the condition may heal itself as the body takes over to compensate for the stroke which led to the optic nerve swelling. There is no treatment. The body must provide its own treatment. I have heard that carrots are good for our eyes. I drank carrot juice early this morning.

There is much to be thankful for. There is much to be concerned about. Those two sentences describe the dual reality which cancer patients face each day, each moment. Perhaps those two sentences describe the dual realities of life itself. Within those two sentences is a life lesson from fighting cancer. Be vigorously thankful for everything you can be thankful for. Be vigorously involved in confronting everything that is of concern.

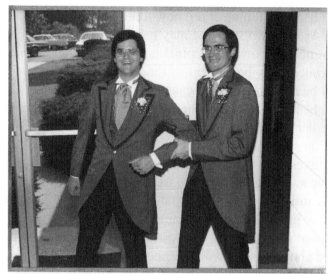

June 9, 1979: Bob and Keen pose for Laura and Bob's wedding
day pictures

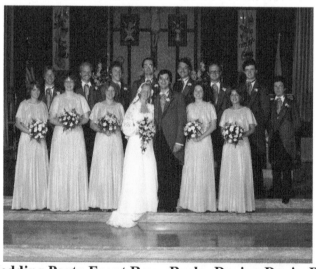

The Wedding Party Front Row: Becky Dusing Davis, Bridget
Bunning Blinn, Cindy Schulte Butcher, Laura Schulte Babbage,
Bob Babbage, Mary Ann Mulcahey, Paula Wade. Back row:
David Schulte, Greg Schulte, Don Cowan, Keen Babbage, Foster
Ockerman, Jr, Jim Dingus, Brad Cowgill, Randy Jedele

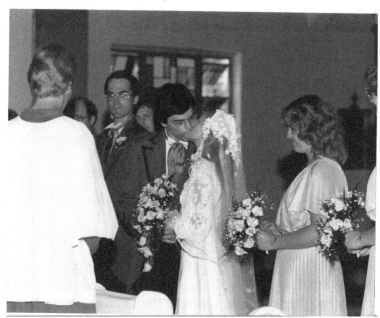

**Keen looks on as Laura and Bob kiss after exchanging vows at St. Joseph Church in Crescent Springs, KY**

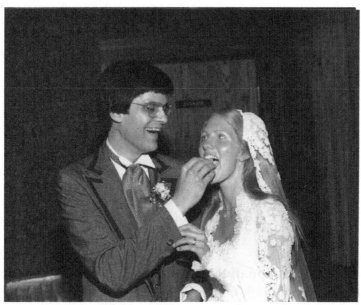

**Laura and Bob at their wedding reception at the Drawbridge Inn in Ft. Mitchell, KY**

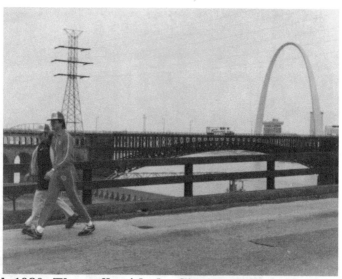

**March 1980: The walk with the Cincinnati Reds Opening Day game ball begins in St. Louis at the headquarters of the manufacturer that provided baseballs for major league teams**

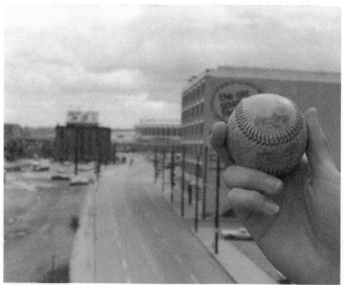

**April 1980: Cincinnati Reds Opening Day baseball arrives in downtown Cincinnati, Ohio after Keen makes the 430-mile trek from St. Louis carrying the baseball**

# Cincinnati Post

Monday evening, March 24, 1980

─focus─

# Fan takes a ball, long walk for Reds

**By Diane Pucin**
*Post Staff Reporter*

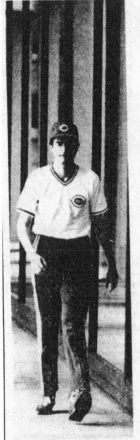

Keen Babbage

In the corporate world of Procter and Gamble—where men and women are garbed in three-piece suits, the carpeted halls are hushed, the security is tight—Keen Babbage is unique.

At work one day last week, Babbage had a suit on. But everyone who passed Babbage in the hall looked at his feet. Because Babbage had on a pair of track shoes—certainly not the look recommended at a major company.

This 25-year-old lifelong Cincinnati Reds fan will be getting his first chance to see an Opening Day game this year. While some people camp out overnight or stand in line for tickets, Babbage is taking a walk for his pass in—430 miles from St. Louis to Riverfront Stadium to be exact.

BABBAGE CAME UP with the most novel way to deliver the first baseball of the 1980 season to Riverfront. He's going to the Rawlings Sporting Goods main office in St. Louis where that first ball is made. And he's going to walk it back to Cincinnati.

The idea had its beginnings when Babbage, who is a volunteer for March of Dimes, was at a meeting to discuss this year's Superwalk—an event where people walk through Cincinnati and collect pledges for the miles they cover.

Someone knew that the Reds were looking for a way to get the first ball delivered (last year it was canoed up the Licking River) and the group decided the walk from St. Louis to Cincinnati would be a good way to promote their Superwalk.

Who would do the walkng? The group considered having members of different March of Dimes chapters along the way take turns, Babbage explained. "But we decided the best way would be to have one person do it."

BABBAGE'S FRIENDS on the group immediately looked at him.

"I thought about it over night. I figured if I took my two weeks vacation I could make it," he said.

A friend will be driving a van to keep Babbage supplied with refreshments. But the physical fitness buff isn't worried at all that he might not make it.

"I've been training for a while now. I quit running and started walking a year or so ago," he said.

"I figure a normal pace is 4 mph and even if I have to slow that down a little if I walk 10 hours a day I can average 30-35 miles a day without a problem.

The trip starts Wednesday morning and is scheduled to end April 9 when Babbage will join the Findlay Market Parade into Riverfront.

"I heard Dick Wagner said that if I was late, they'd start without me so I can't afford a delay," Babbage laughed.

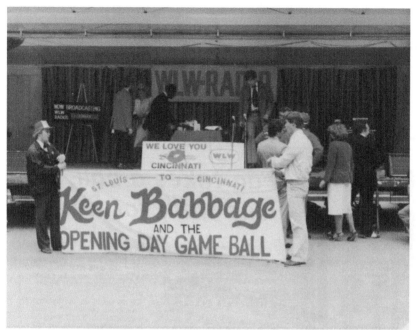

**Fountain Square, Cincinnati, Ohio, Opening Day celebration**

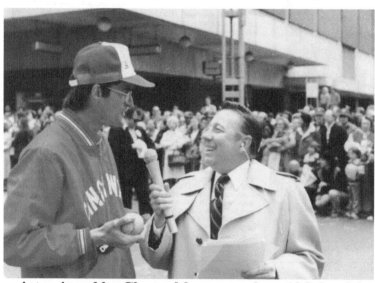

**Keen interviewed by Channel 9 news anchor, Al Schottlekotte during the Opening Day parade**

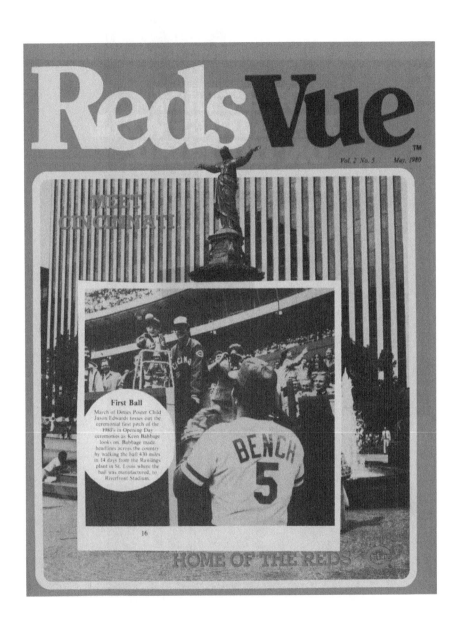

# RedsVue ™

Vol. 2 No. 5.  May, 1980

MEET CINCINNATI

**First Ball**

March of Dimes Poster Child Jason Edwards tosses out the ceremonial first pitch of the 1980's in Opening Day ceremonies as Keen Babbage looks on. Babbage made headlines across the country by walking the ball 430 miles in 14 days from the Rawlings plant in St. Louis where the ball was manufactured, to Riverfront Stadium.

BENCH 5

16

HOME OF THE REDS

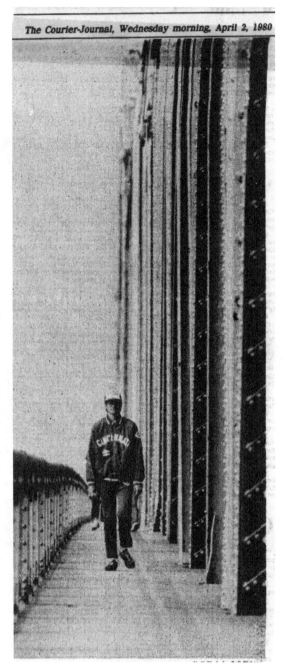

**Keen arrives in Louisville, Kentucky, with the Opening Day game ball**

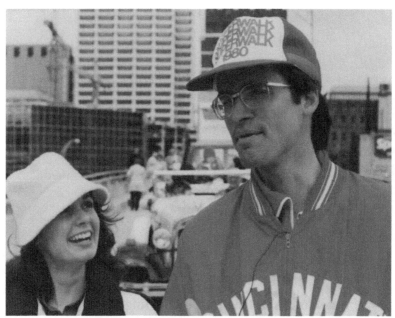

**Lexington, Kentucky *P.M. Magazine* host Lydia Hodson interviews Keen**

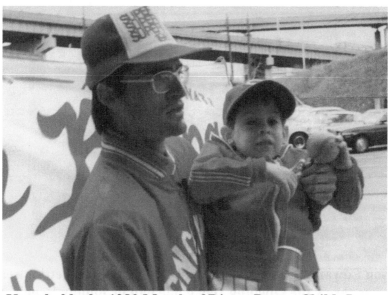

**Keen holds the 1980 March of Dimes Poster Child, Jason Edwards, who holds the Opening Day game ball**

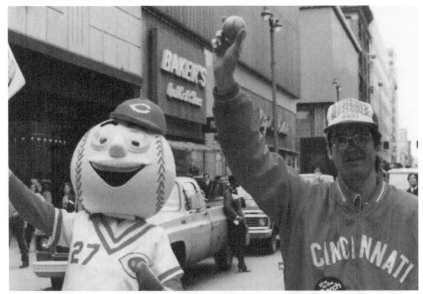

**Keen and Mr. Red in the Opening Day parade**

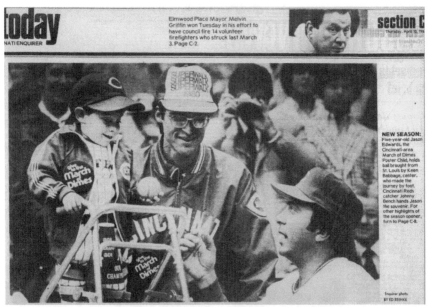

**Jason Edwards, Keen and Johnny Bench. Jason is getting ready to throw the Opening Day game ball to Johnny Bench**

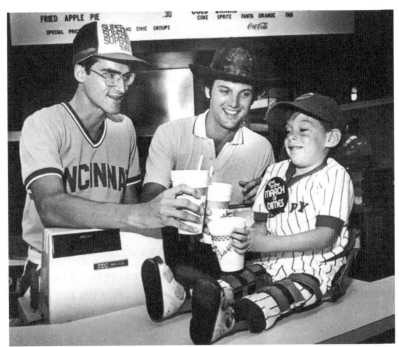

**Fundraiser for the March of Dimes. Keen, Reds player Ron Oester and Jason Edwards**

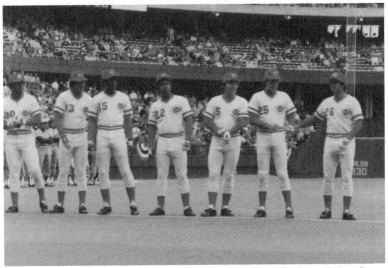

**Opening Day Cincinnati Reds line up for National Anthem**

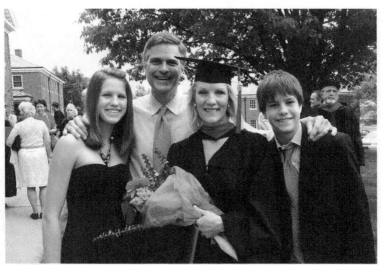

May 11, 2007: Laura graduates from Lexington Theological
Seminary earning her M. Div. She celebrates with her daughter
Julie, husband Bob and younger son Brian. Older son Robert
was away at college

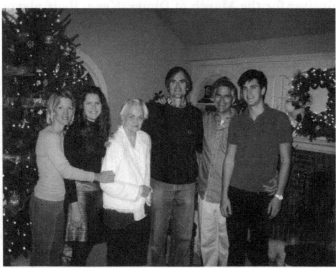

December 13, 2009: The annual Christmas tree decorating at the
Babbages. Nana's last Christmas. From L to R: Laura, Julie,
Nana, Keen, Bob and Robert

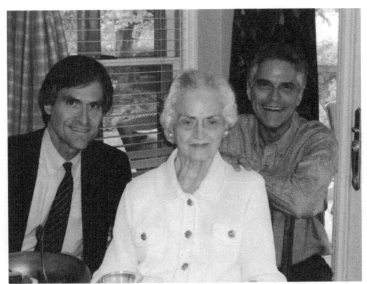

**May 10, 2010: Nana's 83rd birthday party. We had no idea it would be her last**

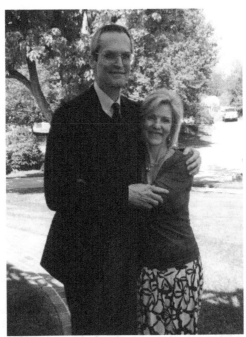

**May 5, 2011: Keen and Laura enjoy a celebratory hug four months after cancer treatments end**

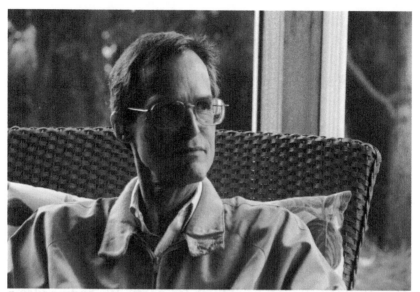

June 11, 2011: Keen in a thoughtful moment on big brother's back porch

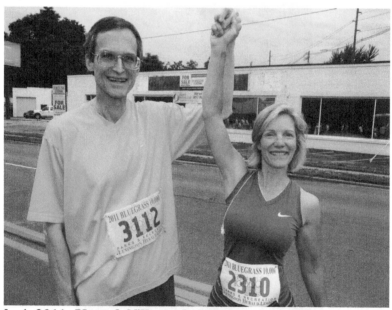

July 4, 2011: Keen fulfills goal of completing a 10K post cancer treatment. Although the pace had slowed to a walk, he and Laura finished together

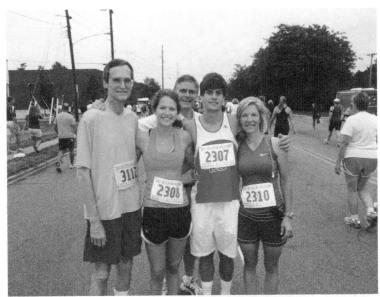

**Keen, Julie, Bob, Brian and Laura pose for a picture before the annual Bluegrass 10,000**

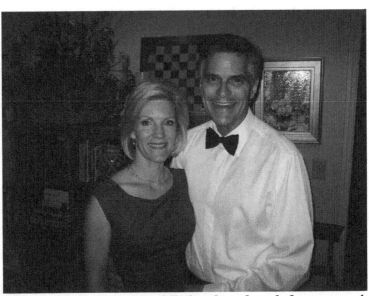

**October 30, 2010: Laura and Bob take a break from caregiving for a night of celebration**

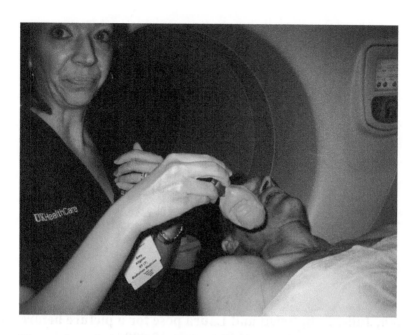

November 4, 2010: Keen about to slide into the radiation machine tunnel while the radiation technician holds the obturator he must put into his mouth

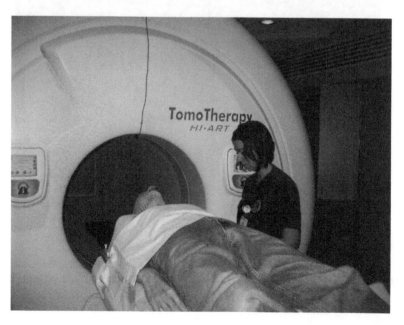

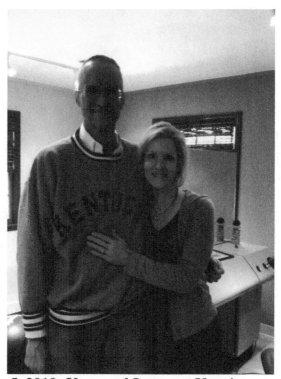

November 5, 2010: Keen and Laura at Keen's second haircut

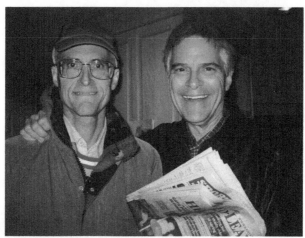

November 6, 2010: Bob takes Keen to chemotherapy prepared with reading material for the treatment at Markey Cancer Center

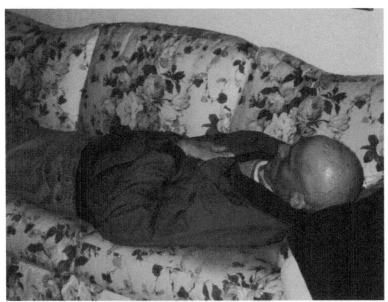

November 20, 2010: Keen rests on the couch at Laura and Bob's house. The cancer treatments are beginning to take their toll on him

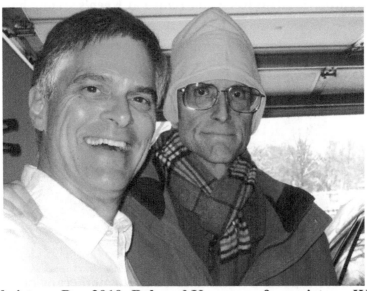

Christmas Day 2010: Bob and Keen pose for a picture. We decided to repeat every holiday in 2011

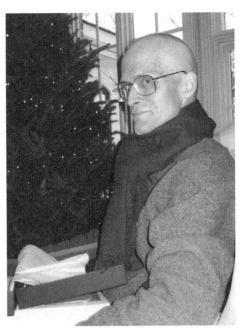

**Christmas Day 2010: Keen demonstrates the proper way to tie a neck scarf**

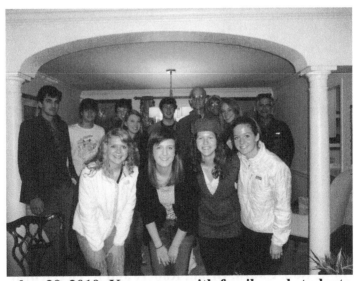

**December 29, 2010: Keen poses with family and students over the Christmas holiday**

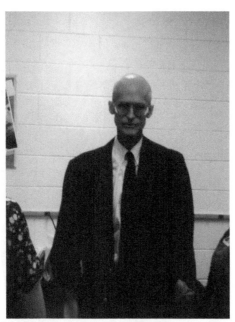

January 28, 2011: Keen returns to the Henry Clay High School
to teach one class period—Political Science. It was a great day

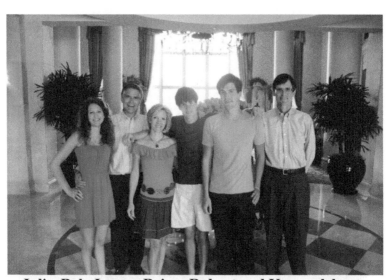

Julie, Bob, Laura, Brian, Robert and Keen celebrate
Thanksgiving in Florida 10 months after cancer treatments
ended, another milestone achieved

# Saturday, January 1, 2011

Keen met his New Years Day goal—*eat a scrambled egg*—check! It was a great start to a new year. Shortly after his cancer treatment began in October, Keen said, "I'd like to sleep through this; wake me up in January." We are there. Radiation is over, and round four of Chemo begins on Tuesday. Although some days are better than others (most are still mediocre at best), Keen continues to battle cancer with energy, hope and determination.

A positive side effect of becoming home-bound is Keen's ability to "text message." As you would expect from the master teacher, his texts are complete with proper punctuation and complete sentences. If you are inspired to do so, send him a text message sometime this month (don't worry, he will not correct your grammar or punctuation).

# Wednesday, Jan 5, 2011

On the way to our second day of round four of chemo, Keen said, "I have endured a grueling 10 day hospital stay, pneumonia, explosive diarrhea, 35 radiation treatments, and three rounds of chemo, and yet the only thing that has brought a tear to my eyes is when I think about my students...it is what I was called to do...I should be teaching my first period political science class right now."

The longing and the sorrow were palpable. We sat silently in the car and looked straight ahead. Tears rolled down Keen's cheek. Then he asks, "How is your family this morning?"

Keen reached a turning point on Monday when he wrote: "Monday, January 3, 7:30 a.m. Enough is enough. I just drank a sip of water. Then I drank another. Two, count 'em. Two sips. As I will tell Dr. Arnold today, I am sick of being sick and tired. Let's win this war against cancer and move on to better living to the Glory of God. Love ya."

And that was that. He took off his grey fleece and sweatpants and put on his new cords and sweater. It is time to get back to living...and that includes getting dressed and eating, driving his car and most importantly, teaching.

This week includes more doctor appointments and recovering from chemo. Next week will be tiring from the effects of chemo. On Jan 18, Keen will have another MRI and CT scan to evaluate the success of treatment. After that, decisions will be made regarding additional treatment. The goal is to get back in the classroom as soon as possible so Keen will look into options to make that possible.

# Saturday, January 8, 2011

Round four of chemo was worse than expected. The healing was beginning on the mouth and throat and now chemo has irritated and worsened that small victory. Keen writes early this morning, "The chemo impact is worse than I anticipated, so I just cope with that and do very little else. It makes me very weary and it complicates mouth/throat conditions. It is a time for much prayer and to ask for new healing."

The impact of notes and visits from family and friends is immeasurable. Thanks for the many ways you continue to remember Keen and our family.

# Monday, January 17, 2011

Tomorrow is the day Keen has his CT scan and MRI. The scans will provide information about the cancer that will determine next steps. Your prayer for a full and complete healing is what we are asking for. Cancer is a roller coaster of emotions. Keen said recently, "I can't imagine not crying on my first day back in the classroom." Of course you will cry, I said, it is the only human response you can have to such an awful thing.

Getting back to "normal" routines has been the goal since Keen shared his diagnosis and treatment plan with his students on October 13, 2010. "We need to help the doctors understand that part of my getting better is getting back to work," Keen said with conviction. A move in that direction is that Keen started driving again two weeks ago. Although he tires in the afternoons, his mornings are full with meetings and errands.

Keen was able to attend church on Sunday, saying, "I went to 8:30 a.m. service this morning. I walked out of my condo at 8:15 and was in the pew at 8:25. It was a wonderful service and it was very encouraging to be there." Oh, I forgot to mention that another very extraordinary but "normal" activity last week was moving to a condo—something Keen had decided to do this summer before his mom became ill and before cancer. Keen's comment to big brother Bob about his new place was, "It felt more like home the first night I was here than all 22 years at my old home." Confirmation of a good decision!

Keen's next goal is to work on swallowing again. He said, "I swallowed some water earlier today with no difficulty. My mouth and throat need much healing, but they are not as awful as they have been...It is time to add to the feeding tube so the day of removing the tube can come sooner, in fact as soon as possible." The scale Keen has developed to explain how he feels when asked by his doctors is: silence and tears, awful, not as awful, ok. We are working up to "good" and "very good." Patience can be a tough virtue to hold on to in the midst of battle.

# Wednesday, January 19, 2011

No results yet on the CT scan and MRI. Keen has a doctor's appt on Friday with his ENT doctor who made the original diagnosis and on Monday with his Radiation and Oncology doctors. We continue to pray.

Yesterday Keen ate a chocolate jello pudding cup. "At least it doesn't taste bad," was his comment. Today it was yogurt for breakfast and a yet to be determined "yummy" for dinner. There are no shortcuts to recovery.

# Monday, January 24, 2011

We hate to complain about the UK "system," but as I drove through the car wash after Keen's appointment today he said, "Maybe they know how to get the MRI results, they seem efficient!" Neither the ENT doctor on Friday nor the radiation doctors today had Keen's MRI results in the computer. "It just doesn't seem that difficult to get," Keen responded.

Tomorrow we meet with Keen's oncologist who will share the results of his scans as well as treatment options from the "team" of doctors who will be discussing his ongoing care at an early morning conference. The oncologist has tentatively scheduled round five of chemotherapy to begin tomorrow, but the final decision has not yet been made.

Keen had an active weekend. He went to his nephew's indoor track meet at UK (Brian ran very well in the 200 and 400 meter race), and then to church twice! "They had a second service devoted to the youth so I went a second time," Keen said with enthusiasm. He also ate three times and reported to his doctors that he had no trouble getting the food down. His goal is keep eating—so eat, eat more, keep eating is our new mantra!

Today after his appointment Keen bought a new microwave and a few other kitchen necessities—like a bowl, wisk, spatula and frying pan. Cooking is new territory for Keen, so he decided to begin with scrambled eggs. After all his questions were answered about techniques for scrambling eggs, he could have written the manual. You can take the teacher out of the classroom but...

# Tuesday, January 25, 2011

"It looks so good that we need to be sure," was the ENT doctors encouraging, hoped for and prayed for words today. "Is it normal? No. Will it ever be? No. We need to clean out what we see in the sinuses, maybe take some biopsies and then re-scan you." Clearly the doctors are encouraged by the treatment results. We are not out of the woods. Keen will have outpatient sinus surgery next Monday. That will provide additional information including whether or not any further Chemo is needed. It will also tell us if other treatment may be necessary. We are grateful and hopeful.

Your prayers, thoughts and constant good wishes are appreciated beyond words. Keen has already prepared some lesson plans, had the tires changed on his car and visited the grocery store for high calorie food. The "new normal" just started looking better. We will take it. In the words of Keen's mom as she prayed with him before she died, "PLEASE, Amen."

# Friday, January 28, 2011

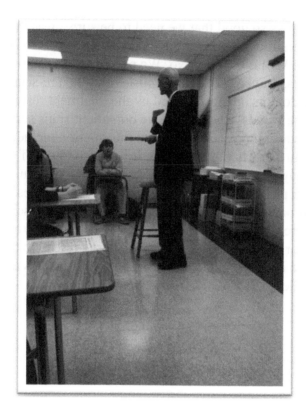

    It was a day to remember at Henry Clay High School. Dr. Babbage arrived this morning well before the first bell and taught his first period political science class. Just like every good sister-in-law would want to know on the first day back in the classroom, I asked, "What are you going to wear?" I asked. Surprised by the question, Keen said, "My suits would fall off of me," and then began thinking about what might work. Dr. Babbage settled on a signature white shirt, grey and black striped tie, blue blazer and grey slacks—he looked great albeit thinner and with just a bit of peach fuzz growing atop his head. He was greeted with tears, smiles, hugs and warm wishes. It was a day he had imagined hundreds of times since sharing his diagnosis with his students on October 13th.

    Keen surprised his first period students with a gift. He gave each student a Lincoln $1 presidential coin explaining that since he received prize money from an essay contest that one of his students had won, he was sharing half his prize money with the class. It is a practice Dr. Babbage is known for at HCHS.

"Thanks be to God for a morning I will remember forever. What a blessing." This was Keen's immediate response to his visit back to school, adding a bit later, "The blessings and inspiration of this morning continue to bless me beyond all I could have asked or imagined."

No one would request a diagnosis like cancer. No one. And yet the ways in which Keen has battled his illness and unfailingly imagined the day he would walk back into the classroom, using his gifts and inspiring students, touches us all. Of course, one class was not quite enough. Keen left his first period classroom, walked confidently down the hallway, pausing from time to time to receive a kind word from a student or well wishes from a fellow teacher, to his second period class where he was greeted with hugs and smiles. "What's the subject?" he asked Mr. Snow, "The Populist Movement," was the answer given. Without missing a beat, Dr. Babbage asked, "What was that Movement a response to?" Mr. Snow took a seat in the back of the classroom while Dr. Babbage, without a note, used his infamous Socratic method to encourage the students to explain the Populist Movement. We all learned together.

It was a very good morning, one that will inspire Keen to eat, eat more and keep eating. He will gain weight, and do what his doctors ask of him. He will be ready for the day when he can return full-time to the classroom.

# Life Lesson: Build a Network and Never Let Go

Dear Dr. Babbage,

We miss you at school. We hope you are getting well. You always tell us to read, read more, keep reading. Our message to you is fight, fight more, keep fighting. We are praying for you.

Sincerely,

Your Students

One of my fondest hopes, one of my most inspiring hopes, one of my most deeply held hopes during the time I had to miss months due to cancer was to return to school.

When you are motivated to get well because other people need you to get well, you are doubly inspired. One inspiration to recover is because you are determined to live more, longer, better. You are not finished with your life's work on earth, so you are urging yourself to get well.

Another inspiration for fighting to recover is that other people long to share part of life with you again. The first motivation—getting well for yourself—is powerful, but has limits. The second motivation—to get well for other people—is more powerful and has no limits.

Work hard to get well for yourself. Work harder to get well for other people. What we do in life for other people evokes a response deep within that surpasses the response we have when our effort is purely for self.

Make the most of the motivation for self. You are eager to be well again and let that eagerness help get you through the difficult days in the cancer war. More can be made of the motivation for others. Fighting the good fight one more day with one more burst of energy that you alone do not have will bring new hope to you and new hope to family and friends.

Let yourself say these words, "I need to get well." True. You do need that, hope for that, seek that, long for that and go through brutal treatments for that.

Now, let yourself say these words as you think of family and friends: "I need to get well for you. I need to get well for us." As you multiply the reasons to get well, you multiply the resolve to get well.

In the war against cancer, you need every possible advantage. You can recruit an anti-cancer team. Cancer cannot recruit an anti-you team. Cancer fights you alone and it fights to kill. Outnumber cancer, overpower cancer with a team that fights, fights more and keeps fighting.

*　　*　　*

Building a network means there is some construction work to do. This construction is done with phone calls, letters, e-mail, text messages, websites and face-to-face conversations. When the words "you have cancer" are heard, one of the early reactions should be the creation of a network which will be part of your anti-cancer army.

Tell people that you have cancer. Many of those people will ask "What could I do to help you?" Tell them specifically what you need them to do. "Please take me to my chemotherapy on Monday and stay with me during those four hours. It really helps to have someone to talk to and someone to read to me."

"Please call every church in town where you know someone. Ask them to have people come visit me when I have chemotherapy treatments. If you could set up that schedule it would help so much. Maybe you could come with me to one treatment."

"I cannot cut the grass anymore. If you or your family could do that it would take that off my mind."

"I have to wear a pain patch while I go through these months of treatment. The pain medication is so strong that I cannot drive. I will need rides to treatment, to doctor appointments, to the grocery, to church. If you could set up a group of available drivers it would help my family a lot. They just can't always drive me all the time."

"I can't always make sense out of these medical bills and statements I get from my insurance company. If you know someone who can explain that to me, it sure would help."

"It's hard for me to keep up with the daily activities at home. My family needs to be fed, but it's not easy for me to cook. I have no appetite and it is unpleasant to cook. Do you know people who could fix suppers for my family? Do you know anyone who could come cook for us and we could just warm-up the food for several days?"

"Just call me. I can't go to work for a few weeks. I'm at home alone a lot. I just need to hear from people. Some people know I have cancer and they may think I need to be alone and quiet and resting. I need to be in touch with people. So phone calls would mean a lot."

"Please come visit me. My children are at school all day. My husband is at work, but he leaves the house later and comes home earlier—his boss is really understanding—but there are many hours when I am by myself. Visits would really help me."

"For some reason it is hard for me to read now. I always read the newspaper. I just can't do that now. Could you help me figure out how to listen to that radio service that has people who volunteer to read the newspaper?"

"I might need to get in touch with cancer support groups. You know people who have had cancer. You used to volunteer with that cancer support group at your church. How can I contact groups like that and go to their meetings?"

"I never understand everything the doctors and nurses tell me. They often speak medical language. I don't know all those fancy words. How can I make sense of all that? Is there anybody you know who can go to the medical appointments with me and be my advocate?"

"You are my family. I need you now more than ever. I'm the one who has cancer, but our whole family is impacted by me having cancer. I don't want you to quit everything you do, but for awhile there may need to be some adjustments. We have always helped each other with everything. All of you have done everything I could ask for since the moment I was diagnosed. We love each other. We're family. We'll fight this cancer together. Our love will be stronger than ever."

Build a network. Cancer patients need a lot of help. Cancer patients may not always realize how much help they need. When I was at the worst moment of my war, thus far, with cancer, a picture of me was taken as I managed to sit up momentarily in the hospital bed. Recall that I saw that picture two years after it was taken. My reaction was, "Who is that?" I thought it was a person one generation older than myself. After some further study I realized that the picture was of me. I had been much sicker than I realized. I had needed much more help than I would have known to ask for.

When friends, family, church pastors or members or hospital chaplains visited me during my 10 days in the hospital it gave me a reason to fight harder. It put me in touch with the parts of life I was otherwise separated from. It gave me hope. It brought life to me in the midst of a potentially deadly condition. Those visits alone could not heal me, but they could and did encourage me, sustain me, renew me and give me a reason to dig deeper into myself and fight harder. Without those visits, the effort to recover would have been much more difficult to maintain.

Be specific. Ask a certain person to do an exact action. "You have a snow blower don't you? My husband is out of town today and our driveway is covered. I know it is a lot to ask, but it would help so much if you could clear off our driveway and sidewalks."

"I can't get myself to the grocery store today or any day for that matter. Could I go with you, please, the next time you need to do grocery shopping?"

Once you establish your network of family, friends and others who are willing to help you in the trench warfare versus cancer, hold onto that network. Keep them informed of good news and of bad news. Some people may be reluctant to call, to visit, to inquire because they do not want to interrupt your rest or because they just do not know what to say to or what to do for a cancer patient. Start the conversation for them. Tell them of the exact help you need.

Make a mental note that if you ever feel better, you will respond to the people who helped you with extra acts of kindness. Those people are not asking to be paid back for the help they provided. Still, look what happens to life itself when people help you and later you do something kind for them which otherwise you would not have done. That means acts of kindness, of help, of love, of caring can multiply. In a world where cancer cases and cancer cells viciously multiply, people of kindness and love must multiply their actions much more. Build a network and never let go.

# Monday, Jan 31, 2011

"He's clean as a whistle...I see no evidence of tumor anywhere," Keen's doctor just reported after surgery. It was the news we have all prayed for over these three long and excruciating months of treatment. "We aren't out of the woods yet...we will follow him closely with scans, but we won't be doing round five of chemo that was scheduled to begin Monday," Dr. Gal reported enthusiastically.

There are no more words right now. We know you share in our joy and thanksgiving. We are grateful beyond words.

# Surgery to Clean Out the Sinus Cavity

Dr. Gal wanted to be sure that the only thing left in Keen's sinus cavity was normal radiated tissue. Nothing is ever "normal" again, that was clear, and Dr. Gal wanted to try and give Keen some relief from the constant nasal congestion. The surgery seemed to go longer than expected. When I asked the receptionist for a second time to check on him she said, "He has been in recovery for an hour, you can go back now."

By the time I got to his cubicle, Keen was ready to get dressed and leave. Dr. Gal had already given us the preliminary report which sparked a spontaneous mini celebration in the recovery room. Although we knew that the tissue that was extracted from the sinus cavity would be sent off to the lab for analysis, we cautiously celebrated.

The nurse helped Keen get dressed. I steadfastly refused to assist in those personal matters. As Keen was dressing, I stood outside the curtained cubicle. "Laura, do you have my wallet and keys?" Keen asked through the curtain. "Yes, of course," I said with just a slight irritation. "Can I have them please?" I suggested he finish dressing and then I would give him his wallet and keys. "Can I have them now?" he asked. "Just finish up and I'll give them to you," I said. "I'd like them now please." "Why do you want them now?" I asked. "It's how I get dressed," he said matter-of-factly. "You need your wallet and keys to put your clothes on?" I asked incredulously and with more than a little irritation in my voice. "Yes, I have a process. I put my wallet and keys in my pocket as I am getting dressed," he said. Later, upon reflection I realized how important these small acts of control are to a cancer patient, especially to one who has managed his life the same way for so many years.

# Wednesday, February 2, 2011

"It is all negative...all negative," Keen said through tears, "Dr. Arnold just called to share the great news," he added. Every tissue sample sent for analysis came back revealing no cancer in the sinus cavity. "On Sunday we will celebrate more than the Super Bowl," Keen said. And so we will. Easter has come early this year.

After many long, dark nights of the soul we celebrate this news with you. Clearly your prayers and good wishes have meant everything, and we will continue to rely on your prayers and support. Keen has an appointment with his ENT doctor on Tuesday followed by an MRI and CT scan. His follow up care will be frequent and thorough. Keen said, "This feeding tube cannot come out soon enough!" It is one remaining reminder of the past, and Keen is ready to orient his life to the present and future. He is already making plans that involve more calories, more activity and getting back to the classroom. There is so much life to be lived.

# Thursday, February 3, 2011

"The feeding tube is out," Keen writes, "OUCH!!" For a guy who almost never uses exclamation points, it must have really hurt. "The peg inside the stomach is about one inch diameter and it has to come through the tiny opening (in the stomach). Quite a shock," he continues, "but only for a few moments." As soon as Keen learned that he didn't need chemo-round five, he called his doctor to firmly request a date for the removal of the feeding tube. Well, that is one more "check" on the list or as Keen writes, "One more step toward being normal again."

Of course, it is a new normal. Nothing is ever quite the same post-cancer (PC) as it was before cancer (BC). We use PC and BC when talking about the food Keen plans to eat and activities he plans to do. "If I ever say I am too busy to play tennis with Brian, tell me, 'Keen, that was before cancer!'" Desserts are now on the "approved" list and spending spring break in Florida walking on the beach and goofing off is also on the list. Personally thanking members at the many churches who have been praying for Keen is at the top of his "to do" list. "I have one sermon I want to preach," Keen says.

Keen has been an inspiration to so many. Last Friday, his first visit back in the classroom, in the midst of the hugs and smiles, Keen received several gifts. A student had a package for Keen—it was a scarf he had knitted. Keen, surprised and grateful accepted it and has not taken it off his neck. Another student shared with Keen that he decided to rededicate himself to becoming a better student saying, "I decided that if you could endure all you have gone through, I could do all I can to become a better student." Another student gave Keen a book and asked, "Is it ok to give you a hug?" Keen accepted the hug with gratitude.

# Life Lesson: Fight. Fight More. Keep Fighting

Is there a place for anger in the war against cancer? Does it help to get mad at cancer?

It is understandable to be angry at cancer. It may be common to become mad at cancer. My question becomes "Does it do the cancer patient any good to be angry at cancer or to get mad at cancer?" A related question is "Does it do the family or the friends of cancer patients any good to be angry with cancer?" I would suggest that such anger is unproductive.

It takes effort to be angry. All the effort and energy of the cancer patient needs to be directed toward fighting cancer. Effort consumed by such anger is lost effort.

Cancer cannot hear you, so if you angrily yell at it the words have no impact on the cancer. Those words are unproductive.

Cancer cannot feel your wrath. If you seek a way to angrily get even with cancer you are setting a goal that distracts you from the real goal which is to fight cancer.

Would it make any sense to get angry at chemotherapy, at radiation, at cancer doctors, at nurses, at medical technicians, at workers in medical offices who schedule appointments? That would be rude, unappreciative and unproductive.

It is completely understandable and fully human to be heartbroken, devastated, shocked and anguished when the cancer diagnosis is spoken to the cancer patient. The emotions that cancer ignites are complex, deep and painful. Experiencing those emotions is normal. Expressing those emotions could be therapeutic, but I would advise putting the least amount of time, energy and effort into anger, being mad or expressing the rage emotions that cancer can ignite.

Put your time, energy and effort into fighting cancer. Being stoic may be excessive, but being logical has merit. "I am sick. I have a disease which seeks to kill me. The disease is very vicious, very evil, very wicked and very relentless. I hate this disease, but anger will not defeat cancer. I am inclined to be angry and to be mad at cancer, at me having cancer, at life for putting me in this situation. I have to face this war with my total concentration, will, resolve, courage and effort. No distractions are allowed. Cancer probably wants me to be angry and mad. Instead I will be bold and powerful."

Anger is understandable and tempting, but anger does not defeat cancer. Do only the actions which can defeat cancer. Cancer benefits if you get angry because anger takes your energy and attention. Give cancer no benefits. Give cancer a series of endless, relentless attacks.

*    *    *

My voice broke. I was halfway through a sentence and the next word would not come out of my mouth. I said softly to myself, "Come on, Dr. Babbage, talk."

With about three minutes left in my first period political science class on Wednesday, October 13, 2010 I said the following:

"Now we need to talk about the next few months." So far there was nothing alarming in the concluding comments for the day.

"I will have to miss school until January or February. We don't know....." and then my usually certain classroom speaking ability failed me. The room had become extremely quiet. I had taught some of these students the previous year in U.S. History classes so we knew each other well.

"We don't know exactly when I will return. I was told yesterday that I have cancer, sinus cancer. The treatments will begin tomorrow. I encourage you to keep working and learning. As always, read, read more, keep reading."

There was a very capable substitute teacher in my classroom for this day. I would have to leave at 9:30 a.m. for meetings with doctors who would be involved with my treatments. The substitute asked, "Dr. Babbage, do they know much about your condition?"

I explained that no cause of the sinus cancer was known. I told her and the class that I would have chemotherapy and radiation therapy. Then the bell rang to end class.

Several students were quite slow to leave the classroom. Their encouraging comments to me, pats on my back or handshakes were genuine and were appreciated.

What goes through the mind of a 17-year-old high school student whose teacher just announced that for the next four months cancer treatments would force the teacher who never misses school to miss a lot of school?

Perhaps they wondered why I would be gone so long. Perhaps they wondered if I would ever return. Perhaps they wondered if I would die of cancer.

About 20 students made extra effort to encourage me in the war against cancer. They wrote letters. They sent e-mails. They attended study sessions with me. They prayed for me. They brought gifts.

I was determined to return and to finish the school year with those students and the 100 others in my five classes. Being away from them meant I was sick. Being back with them meant cancer lost.

Their vibrant teenage lives would continue. They would advance in their senior or junior year of high school. They would keep learning about U.S. History and Political Science without me. I would learn about cancer, chemotherapy, radiation, side effects, the realistic possibility of death and the endless power of faith, family and friends.

Being back with the students was an inspiring reason to fight, fight more, keep fighting. The cancer patient needs incentives such as that.

There are times when the desire to not die is an insufficient incentive. The desire to live as fully as possible must endure. For me, part of living fully would include getting back to school. The hope for that return, the need for that return, the determination for that return added vigor when I was weary and purpose when I was perplexed.

On my first day working again at school—Monday, February 28, 2011—my voice did not break. I did not look like myself due to no hair and 35 pounds less, but as always I wore a suit. Students who might not recognize me with a different appearance would recognize the teacher who always wore a suit. I just worked a half day, but it was so encouraging.

We were together again. I had hoped to be back by January or February and had returned on the last day of February. You lose cancer.

Sunday, February 27 was a unique day. On this afternoon high school seniors in the school district where I teach would pay tribute to the teacher that had made the biggest contribution to their education. During my four recent years of teaching high school, 2006 to 2010, I had been honored by four high school seniors for these teacher recognition awards. One year, three seniors had honored me. Another year, one senior had honored me. Four such awards surpassed any reasonable hope or expectation.

On Sunday, February 27, 2011, four more high school seniors reflected about Dr. Babbage and the meaningful experiences we had shared in the classroom. They joined about 70 other high school seniors who were honoring devoted teachers. I well recall the words spoken by one of my students as he spoke of his junior and senior years of high school in my U.S. History and Political Science classes. That young scholar ended his tribute to me by saying of Dr. Babbage, "He inspires me."

That student was in my classroom on Wednesday, October 13, 2010 when my voice broke as I forced myself to push words out of my mouth. This young scholar's confident and sincere voice was clear. "He inspires me."

As I anticipated returning to school the next day, it was quite true that this student and the three others who chose me as their best teacher were inspiring me. On the next day I would teach again. On the next day part of life as it was before cancer would return to what it had been before cancer.

Many parts of life had changed due to cancer. My return to teaching would be only for half days during the first week. I did not look or feel as I did before cancer.

But if I would walk back into that classroom and begin doing my job again, that would be an epic triumph. The four students whose minds I had sought to touch in our classroom, had, through their actions to honor me, touched my heart, soul and mind. My body was encouraged also.

What the first day back in the classroom would be like could not yet be known, but the fact that it would happen meant that cancer had been denied the power of removing me forever from my chosen profession. I would return to the classroom with limited energy, with a bald head, with 35 pounds removed from my skinny body. I would return to the classroom with the certainty that cancer had lost this part of the war. There were students to teach. There was work to do. There was a strong reminder of why it was, is and would be vital to fight, fight more, keep fighting in the forever war against cancer.

*     *     *

Cancer acts alone its war against you, unless you give cancer some allies. Make cancer fight by itself.

Cancer would like a large group of allies. Cancer wants you to be afraid, absolutely paralyzed, terrorized and controlled by fear. Cancer alone can kill. Cancer plus fear are more likely to kill than is cancer by itself.

How does cancer get to add fear to the cancer axis of evil? By the cancer patient being afraid of cancer instead of being relentlessly combative against cancer.

Isn't cancer scary? Of course. Cancer is life threatening. Cancer is potentially deadly. How can fear be avoided when a person is told that he or she has cancer? Think. Does a cancerous tumor shrink because the cancer patient is fearful? No. Does the chemotherapy have fewer side effects because the cancer patient is fearful? No. Does the radiation treatment have fewer side effects because the cancer patient is fearful? No.

Would not being afraid cause the cancerous tumor to shrink? No. Would not being afraid cause fewer side effects from chemotherapy or from radiation treatments? No. Then what are the benefits of being brave, bold, confident and courageous instead of being fearful, terrified and in a pure panic?

Cancer acts to kill you. It wants to kill your body. While cancer works to kill your body it also would like to defeat your heart, mind and soul.

Remember, the only war cancer can start is the physical war. Cancer viciously attacks the body. Cancer cannot attack the human heart, mind and soul unless the human cancer patient lets cancer do that.

Cancer, you seek to kill my body. Everything possible will be done to kill you before you kill me.

Cancer, you will have no real impact on what I think, what I believe or the type of person I am. As a human, I will have an occasional moment of despair or doubt, of anguish or anxiety, of crisis or emergency, but those moments will not linger. I will realize them for what they are. They are part of your deceptive, evil, wicked mind games.

Cancer, you will score no points in the competition for my heart, my mind or my soul. You are wasting your effort in that competition.

Cancer, you are a physical reality, a physical force and a physical enemy. I will never let you be more than that. I will fight you physically. That is the one and only way you can fight me.

I also will fight you with all my heart, all my mind and all my soul. Cancer, you have none of those. Cancer, you have no heart, mind or soul. And I will never let you have any part of my heart, mind or soul.

You are a thief, cancer. You are stealing some of my physical health. You are stealing some of my time. You will not steal any of my heart, mind or soul.

The part of my physical health which you steal, I will compensate for by maximizing what I achieve through the physical health I still have.

The part of my time which you steal, I will compensate for by maximizing what I can achieve through the time I have every day.

You will get no part of my heart, mind or soul. None. But just to gain an advantage against you, I will increase the quality of, the productivity from and the results from my heart, mind and soul.

Cancer, you picked the wrong fight, at the wrong time, at the wrong place, with the wrong person. Cancer, you lose.

# Friday, Feb 11, 2011

Life does go on...gratefully! Keen taught his political science class recently and visited his second and third period US History classes. He plans to return to school part-time at the end of the month and see how that goes. He is anxious but realistic, another reality of cancer. Some of his teaching methods will change—out of necessity. There will not be any more 80 hour work weeks, Keen's typical schedule before cancer. "There are many ways to be effective in less time," Keen admits.

On Tuesday Keen had his one week post surgery follow up with his ENT doctor. The process of removing some of the remaining nasal packing left Keen groaning in pain and physically exhausted. At one point Keen asked the doctor, "Can you stop for a minute?" and he did. Later as we talked about all his body has endured—35 grueling radiation treatments and four rounds of deadly chemotherapy, dozens of IV's and seemingly endless needle sticks, 10 days at Markey Cancer Center including the insertion of a feeding tube, CT and MRI scans, doctor appointments—we marveled at the capacity of the human body to endure such continuous assault. "We have an extensive prayer network," Keen explains as he talks about his life over the past four months, "that extends beyond Kentucky!" Prayer has been and will continue to be what sustains us in this fight.

The MRI Keen had earlier in the week shows an area of interest that the doctors will continue to watch. After cancer and radiation, the tissue is never "normal" again. Frequent scans will provide a more complete picture and indicate if additional treatment is necessary.

And so it goes, one small step every day. Adjusting to a new normal is never easy—like awakening at night to a mouth so dry that the thirst cannot be easily quenched (the salivary glands were dried up with radiation) and eating food out of necessity even though it no longer has any taste—just the memory of how good it used to be. Keen's response to the changes is, "We haven't finished praying about that yet!"

# Friday, February 25, 2011

Good news! Keen returns part time to the classroom on Monday! If all goes well he will be full-time in another week. It is miraculous and we attribute so much of his healing to you—our ever present, ever prayerful support team.

Now I have another request. Bob (Keen's brother and my husband) discovered last night that he has a detached retina in his right eye. "Just bad luck," the doctor said. He is having a procedure done this morning that we hope will save the vision in his eye. Your prayers and good thoughts mean everything. We will know by Monday if the procedure worked. If not he will have surgery Monday morning. Oh my.

# Saturday, February 26, 2011

It must have been a sight to see. The tall, nearly bald recovering cancer patient walking his shorter nearly blind big brother into the eye clinic while I was home sick with some bad bug. The prayer Keen prayed before he and Bob left must have had the apostles cheering. His confidence in what all "the great physicians" can do is awe-inspiring.

Keen's faith has never wavered. In the depths of the valley of the shadow of death he believed he would be back in the classroom—and now he will be. "I have all my lesson plans for March complete, I am ready," Keen announced with his usual enthusiasm. He's back!

As for Bob, the "bubble" procedure is doing its work and the doctors will laser the retina on Monday. He avoided surgery at least for now but recovery will be slow.

# Tuesday, March 1, 2011

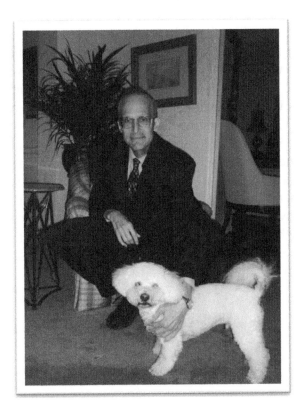

    Great news! The "bubble" procedure worked and Bob's retina re-attached. No surgery required. We are elated and grateful. It is good to have that behind us.

    Keen's first day back at school was everything he had hoped. He arrived early yesterday on a rainy bleak Monday morning to be greeted by excited faculty, staff and students who had been awaiting this day almost as much as he has. His spirits were lifted even higher by the Sunday afternoon "Fame" awards where he was selected by four senior students as the "teacher who has made the biggest difference in my life. You can view the awards by visiting http://www.fcps.net/news/features/2010-11/fame-awards. This ceremony is perhaps the most gratifying of all awards for a teacher. And to be selected by four seniors in one year is even more special.

Keen left for the ceremony, dressed in his "school uniform," a dark navy suit, blue shirt and a tie. He came by the house to check on Bob and our dog Rudy before leaving. "Take good care of yourself, Bro, and get better soon," Keen said as he was leaving. It is something Bob would have said to Keen just a few months ago.

After the program, Keen called us to read one of the papers a former student had written about him. As he read, Bob wept tears of joy and pride for his baby brother. It was quite a moment between two brothers who have shared so much loss and sorrow over the past five months. This was a moment of true celebration.

We continue to fight the battle and pray daily that Keen's cancer will not return. In the meantime, life goes on. There are papers to grade and lesson plans to tweak, encouraging words to offer to students and plans to be made for the future. We hold each of you closely in our prayers and hope that you feel our deep gratitude for being with us throughout these often dark and grueling days of cancer and recovery. Keen's next MRI and CT scan is scheduled for Spring Break week—early April.

# Life Lesson: Ask Many Questions

Ask many questions. Ask. Ask more. Keep asking. In the realm of medical science are many capable, honorable, caring, hardworking people who devote their careers to fighting cancer. Their knowledge, advice, expertise and experience are available to guide, direct and inform you. Ask them every possible question. You deserve to know everything that can be known.

To their credit, healthcare professionals speak the precise language of medical science. That language has a very exact vocabulary which is fully known to people who have been trained in and taught about healthcare. Within the overall vocabulary of healthcare and of medical science is the specific language related to cancer. To the cancer patients, this vocabulary is new. To the family and friends of the cancer patient, this vocabulary is new. Always ask every possible question.

"We need to begin our chemotherapy on Thursday. It will be three consecutive days. You will have a three-day sequence once every three weeks." That statement from a cancer physician to a cancer patient raises many questions.

"Will it hurt?"

"How long does each treatment last?"

"What exactly is chemotherapy?"

"Does the chemotherapy material stay in my body or does it get removed?"

"What will I feel?"

"How does the chemotherapy know where the cancer is?"

"Does the chemotherapy attack only the cancer or does it attack everything?"

"Does this do more good than harm?"

"Are there any other options?"

"What makes this the best action to take?"

"How will we know if it is working?"

"Will it make me sick?"

"Will you be there when I get chemotherapy?"

"What can go wrong?"

"I've heard that chemotherapy has poison in it. Is that true?"

"Will I still be able to go to work on the days I have chemotherapy? What about on the weeks between each three-day session. Can I work then?"

"What am I allowed to do during the chemotherapy treatments? Do I just sit there?"

"Does chemotherapy help most people?"

"Why does chemotherapy make people lose their hair?"

"What are the side effects?"

"How many of these three-day sessions will I need?"

"Can this make me worse?"

"What exactly is in chemotherapy? Is it like any other medicine?"

"What makes the chemotherapy work?"

"What happens if my body just rejects this?"

"Today is Tuesday. We're starting this on Thursday. That does not give us much time to get ready. What happens if I wait?"

"To be honest, this scares me a bit. What am I supposed to do about that?"

"Will chemotherapy make me weak? I've seen people who were on chemotherapy. They look awful. Will I look awful?"

"Why does chemotherapy make people throw up? Is there any way to prevent that?"

"Can I still eat after I start chemotherapy?"

"Does being on chemotherapy make it more likely that I will get sick from something else?"

"Do I have to wear one of those breathing masks everywhere I go?"

"When will this be over?"

"Can you give me a book about chemotherapy? I'd like to know the science of this and the history of this."

"How reliable is chemotherapy? Does it usually work? Is there anything better?"

"What can go wrong?"

"Can my family be with me when I'm getting chemotherapy?"

"Will my insurance pay for all of this chemotherapy?"

"Can I drive myself to chemotherapy or does someone else have to bring me?"

"If you were me is this what you would do? Would you do this chemotherapy to yourself or your family?"

There will be many meetings with doctors. There will be many interactions with nurses, physician's assistants, nurse practitioners, medical technicians, medical appointment schedulers, medical office workers, home health providers and other people in the large world of fighting cancer.

Ask every question you have to every person who deals with you. They know a lot. You need to know what they know. They deal with cancer in general and with many individual cancer patients. You are dealing with the specific cancer that is attacking your body. Work with all of the health care providers to together become experts in your cancer, to together take your cancer personally as if they are the patient as much as you are.

Asking questions informs you. Getting answers equips you. Interacting in the question and answer process helps build the mutual connection which is an essential part of your network of soldiers in the army you have available to fight cancer.

The health care experts will benefit from answering your questions. It gives them new opportunities to think through the many issues, facts, concerns and topics related to fighting cancer. Your questions help the medical experts become better experts. Their answers help you become a strong warrior. Ask. Ask more. Keep asking.

Talk to people who have been treated for cancer. Talk to cancer survivors who are at various points past their last treatment. Talk to family members of current cancer patients. Ask these people what questions they have thought of that they would have asked if they knew earlier what they know now. Some possible questions which come only from experience could include the following among others:

"Once we eliminate the cancer, how long will it take my body to recover from the ordeal the treatments will put me through?"

"Am I going to need surgeries after these treatments because of side effects?"

"In two years after treatments, what will I notice? Will I be back to normal? Will I be getting closer to normal? Will I never be like I was before and just have to realize that normal is impossible?"

"Will I have to keep seeing doctors for the rest of my life as often as I am now? Does that ever slow down?"

"What can I do to keep the cancer from coming back?"

"When I get sick, how will I know if it has something to do with having had cancer and cancer treatments or if it's just regular illness?"

"After a year or two or three, will my fitness level return? These treatments can make people very weak and tired. Is that permanent?"

"I'm used to working 70 hours each week. Will I be able to do that or not?"

"Is it true that radiation causes cataracts? Will I need cataract surgery after these treatments?"

"I have always exercised a lot. I get an hour of exercise five or six days each week. Will I be able to exercise like that again?"

"I have no appetite since these treatments began. Will that change?"

"What am I going to notice year after year once the treatments end? What new side effects and complications are going to appear that are not showing up yet?"

"Once I'm a cancer patient am I always a cancer patient? Will there ever be a day when all of this is over?"

"OK. It's three years after my treatments ended. I've been in remission for three years. I feel something strange. How seriously do I react to each new ache or pain or other change in my body?"

"Tell me why this schedule of treatments is the best for me. Are there options that could be just as effective, but not so brutal?"

"What are the exact chances of someone my age getting well and then getting cancer again?"

"Are these treatments going to make it more likely that I get other sicknesses later on?"

"Is this cancer going to kill me?"

"I heard that chemotherapy hurts hearing. Will I need hearing aids after this?"

Cancer changes your life, forever. Ask questions that deal with the issues of today, of tomorrow, of the near future and of the far future. One way to help take control of the war against cancer is by being 100 percent informed. Ask questions. Ask doctors, nurses, technicians, support group members, family and friends. Read articles, books and websites. Learn. Know. Ask. Fight.

Asking questions is part of fighting cancer. The more questions you ask the more you know about the war you are in. Fully know the enemy. Cancer is the enemy. Fighting cancer is complex and rugged. Equip yourself with the armor of full knowledge. Attend cancer patient/family support groups if that is helpful for you.

You never need to apologize for asking. It is your right and your duty to ask. Insist on complete, real answers. Be armed with the truth, the facts, the insights, the knowledge about cancer so you know the enemy better than you have ever known anything. Why? Because this enemy acts to kill you. You have to outsmart a murderer. That is not how most people usually think. It is how cancer patients must think.

*    *    *

Who would think to ask these questions?

1. Will I have frequent nosebleeds when the treatments are over?
2. Will I lose some hearing due to the treatments? Will I have to buy hearing aids and always wear them?
3. When the treatments are over, will I wake up during the night because my mouth and throat are completely dry?
4. For the rest of my life, will globs of mucus get stuck in my throat and will I have to forcefully cough them out?
5. Will these treatments destroy my tear ducts and cause me to look like I am crying all the time?
6. Will I be so fatigued for years to come that I go to bed at 7:00 p.m. or 8:00 p.m.?
7. How much of my senses of taste and of smell will be lost? Will any of that ever return?
8. Is my energy level going to be low always?
9. Will my strength ever return?
10. Will I have persistent headaches in the years following treatment?
11. When you tell me that the tests are now showing no signs of cancer, does that mean I am well? Does that mean there

could be cancer, but the tests did not detect it? Does it mean I am cured or is the word cured never used?

12. Are the ingredients in chemotherapy poison? Are they toxic? Are you going to make me sicker with these treatments before I get less sick?

13. To get at the tumor, was permanent damage done to nearby healthy tissue by the radiation?

14. To get at the part of the tumor that had entered my brain, was damage done to my brain by that radiation?

15. Will the previously healthy tissue that was scarred by the radiation ever heal?

Ask. Ask more. Keep asking. Know all you can. Learn all you can. Share your new knowledge with other people who are fighting cancer. We are in this together. It is the only way to win.

# Monday, April 18, 2011

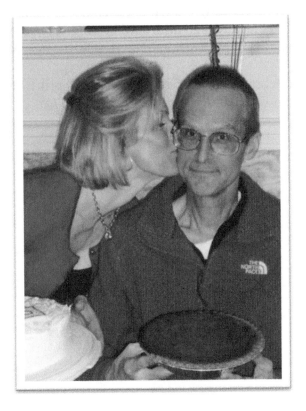

It was a day every mother dares to hope for after a season of trial. Both of Judy's boys had excellent doctor reports today. Keen's cancer is officially in remission and Bob was told by his retina doctor, "don't come back...you're fine." Nana made no secret of the fact that she often prayed that God would never test her faith with her children. In her last days, as she prayed with Keen from her hospital bed for "something important," all Keen asked of his mom was to respond with "Amen" at the end of his prayer.

Today we offer our own prayer of thanksgiving, not only for the remission of cancer and a healed retina, but for you, all of you who have prayed and continue to pray for healing and health with the same determination as Nana. You are never far from our thoughts and prayers as we gratefully thank God for you each time we pray.

We will continue to keep you updated on Keen's progress and healing. He will undergo an MRI and CT scan every three months or more frequently if anything changes. His hair continues to grow back—an outward sign of inward healing, and before long he will go for his first post cancer haircut. It will be cause for more celebration.

We celebrated Keen's 57th birthday on April 1 (no joke) and when asked how he felt, Keen said, "older than 57."

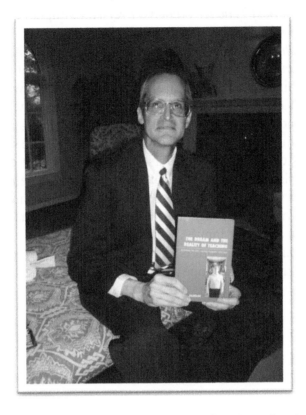

Keen's 13th and by his own declaration, "my last book," has been published. The book is dedicated to Nana: "To Judith Keen Johnson Babbage, my mother and best teacher." In his acknowledgements Keen writes, "This book is dedicated to my beloved mother. Two weeks before my mother died in October 2010, I told her that this book would be dedicated to her. She was very pleased with the dedication, yet as a proud mother she was more pleased that her son had completed another book. She was and she will always be our family's best teacher of faith, of love, and of life. My mother made straight-A grades in every class during her college years in the 1940s at the University of Kentucky. She still holds the family grade-point championship."

The devotion of son to mother was evident not only in words, but in deeds. As Nana's health declined over the years, Keen redoubled his helping efforts. He and Bob were truly devoted sons.

Keen's book, titled *The Dream and Reality of Teaching: Becoming the Best Teacher Students Ever Had*, might have been called, *What I Learned From my Mother at the Kitchen Table: A Master Teacher Shares a Lifetime of Lessons Learned*. Keen writes the way he teaches, with passion, hope and a deep belief that the goal of teaching is to "cause learning to happen," and "we know how to do that," Keen says. Every page of his book is filled with stories, examples, and "how to's" that will have the most unimaginative of teachers taking another look at how to make his/her classroom come alive. Check out the book for yourself at rowmaneducation.com.

As this school year begins the final push to the end, we look back and marvel at all that has been accomplished—so many endings and new beginnings for our family. Surely it has been the same for you and your family. You have been there for us and with us, a community of supporters and pray-ers, many of whom we haven't met and yet who hope and pray with and for us.

# Postscript

Keen's 13th book was not his last, how could it be? His 14th, 15th and 16th books have all been published post-cancer diagnosis and treatment. Some of the decisions that are made in the midst of cancer treatment and recovery are not the ones that stick. Keen was born to write and teach. He will always have a story on his heart and a lesson plan in his mind. This is the story that has consumed the better part of the last two years of his life and ours and it is still a work in process. Keen has good days and worse days, but no great days. He constantly battles the effects of radiation that never fully disappear; they just morph into a new "normal." Keen rejects the term new normal always reminding the doctors, "Nothing about this is normal."

Keen's mind is as sharp as ever and he lives life to the fullest, albeit with less energy and more doctor appointments. As a frequent patient at all his physician offices, Keen is determined to find and treat any possible symptom before it becomes a problem. Many of the questions he asks his doctors are included in this book, and should be part of every patient's manual for fighting the battle against cancer. Just as he does in the classroom, Keen tries to anticipate every possible scenario and then perform his own cross examination of the physicians, nurses, technicians and support staff that care for him. He does not stop until every question has been answered to his satisfaction. Keen is a well-informed consumer who knows the value of asking good questions.

This book is our effort to share the story of patient and caregiver at the most personal level with hope that it might help another family as they suffer through and survive a diagnosis like cancer. It is also a tribute to all the health care professionals and friends who cared for Keen and our family throughout diagnosis and treatment, and who have continued to support us through remission and beyond. We remain grateful for so many blessings.

Laura Babbage, BSN, MA, MDiv
August 2013

# Keen's Acknowledgements

My family did everything possible for me during the life-threatening months of October 2010 to January 2011. My brother, Bob; my sister-in-law, Laura; my nephews Robert and Brian; my niece, Julie; all were angelic. They opened their hearts, home and schedules to make my war with cancer the family's top priority. They and their beloved dog, Rudy, are six vital allies in my war against cancer. They helped guide me through "the valley of the shadow of death" (Psalm 23).

The people at the Markey Cancer Center at the University of Kentucky are exemplary healthcare professionals. The University of Kentucky hospital system has been completely helpful, caring, and supportive. Thanks to Dr. Susanne Arnold, Dr. Thomas Gal, Dr. Mahesh Kudrimoti, and Dr. Marcus Randall all of whom are with the Markey Cancer Center. Thanks also to Dr. Raven Piercey at the University of Kentucky Department of Behavioral Science.

Friends prayed for me, visited me, wrote to me, ran errands for me and helped build a vast prayer network to support me. Their help was crucial.

Some dear high school students whom I taught visited me, wrote to me and encouraged me. Their eagerness for me to return to teaching was inspiring. Many colleagues at school were supportive, kind and caring.

Faith has been essential in my war against cancer. Pastors visited me. Church members visited me. Many churches put my name on their prayer lists. The peace, power and presence of God, sought through those prayers, became the foundation of this war against cancer.

Creating a book is a demanding and fascinating adventure. Adam Turner did masterful work to take the words and pages of this manuscript and create a wonderful book. His creativity and work ethic are exemplary. Cindy Henderson has typed all of the books I have written or co-authored. Her expertise in taking my handwriting and turning it into accurate word-processing is quite a skill.

Keen Babbage, Ed. D.

# Laura's Acknowledgements

Our family is deeply grateful to the physicians who not only diagnosed and treated Keen's cancer, but listened intently to our questions, patiently and honestly answering each question at every visit. Keen's team of physicians willingly made changes to the treatment plan when needed, recognizing those times when the emotional toll of treatment trumped the charted course for treatment.

Dr. Susanne Arnold, oncology specialist, took a personal interest in Keen's care. She has been a family friend for many years. Her immense knowledge of cancer care and chemotherapy, coupled with her gentle and kind ways made all the difference as Keen progressed through his four cycles of chemotherapy. Dr. Thomas Gal, an Ear, Nose and Throat specialist was always efficient and proactive in his treatment. He helped manage and treat all the complications in Keen's nose, eyes and face from 35 radiation treatments that were necessary to kill his cancer. Dr. Mahesh Kudrimoti, developed the targeted plan for radiation treatment. The precision required for the targeted radiation beams were crucial if Keen was to retain his eyesight, taste buds and even his brain function.

I met Dr. Marcus Randall, Chairman of the Department of Radiation Medicine in November 2009 on a flight from Lexington to Charlotte. We were seatmates on that flight when I learned about his work in Radiation Oncology at the University of Kentucky. Little did I know that less than one year later he would become deeply involved in our family. His constant encouragement and unwavering support of Keen and our family throughout Keen's treatment was an unexpected gift.

And to so many others staff members, from nurses to patient transporters, from housekeepers to nursing assistants, from radiation technicians to receptionists, who helped make Keen's treatment bearable, we are grateful.

There were also dear friends who took turns staying with Keen during his hospital stay, prepared "yummy" food for Keen to eat and sent text messages, notes, cards and letters that were uplifting and timely. Thank you.

To the students and prayer partners, some of whom are pictured in this book, who provided regular doses of diversion from the day to day drama of cancer treatments, without all of you, we could not have endured.

Most importantly to my husband Bob who read all the drafts of this book and offered invaluable insights. After 34 years of marriage, I love you more today than the day we said, "I do." And to our three children, Robert, Julie and Brian. You not only loved me through your own suffering during the uncertain and difficult days of your uncle's cancer treatment, but encouraged me and gave me strength to be the primary caregiver for Keen during his treatment. It has been my life's greatest joy to be your mom.

Laura Babbage, BSN, MA, MDiv

# About the Authors

Keen J. Babbage has 29 years of experience as a teacher and administrator in middle school, high school, college and graduate school.

He is the author of *911: The School Administrator's Guide to Crisis Management* (1996), *Meetings for School-Based Decision Making* (1997), *High-Impact Teaching: Overcoming Student Apathy* (1998), *Extreme Teaching* (2002), *Extreme Learning* (2004), *Extreme Students* (2005), *Results-Driven Teaching: Teach So Well That Every Student Learns* (2006), *Extreme Economics* (2007, 2009), *What Only Teachers Know about Education* (2008), *Extreme Writing* (2010), *The Extreme Principle* (2010), *The Dream and Reality of Teaching* (2011), *Reform Doesn't Work* (2012), *The Power of Middle School* (2012) and *Teachers Know What Works: Experience, Not Statistics, Confirms What Will Work* (2013).

Laura Babbage is a perpetual student with a passion for education. Laura earned an undergraduate degree in Nursing from Eastern Kentucky University, an MA from the University of Kentucky Patterson School in International Business and Diplomacy and a Master of Divinity degree from Lexington Theological Seminary.

After working briefly as a bedside nurse, Laura began her career in health care administration, spending 11 years as CEO of the Urgent Treatment Centers, growing the operation from one center in Lexington to multiple sites in Lexington and surrounding counties. Upon completing her seminary education, Laura began her third career working as a hospital chaplain. She currently works at the University of Kentucky Medical Center and St. Joseph Hospital where she provides spiritual and pastoral care to patients and families.

Since she arrived in Lexington in 1979, Laura has taken significant civic leadership roles including chair of the annual campaign for the United Way of the Bluegrass and chair of the Salvation Army board of directors. She is one of the seven co-founders of Leadership Kentucky which celebrated its 25th anniversary in 2010. With a passion for adventure and travel, Laura climbed Mt. Kilimanjaro with her older son in 2010. She is also an avid cyclist.

Laura is married to Bob Babbage who heads Babbage Cofounder. They have three children, Robert, Julie and Brian.

# Check out these other great titles!

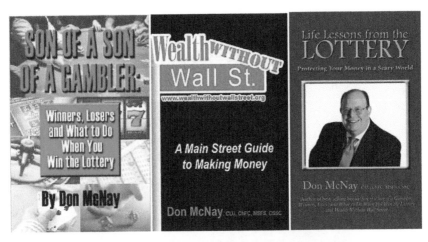

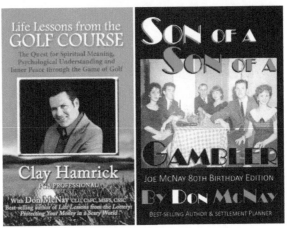

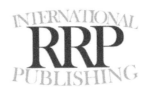

CPSIA information can be obtained at www.ICGtesting.com
Printed in the USA
LVOW02*0851060913

351269LV00001B/1/P